Shallow Dive

Essays on the Craft of Manual Care

Beth,
For the heart
of your own
Practice
Barrett 1/21/96

Shallow Dive

Essays on the Craft of Manual Care

Barrett L. Dorko, PT
Cuyahoga Falls Physical Therapy
Cuyahoga Falls, Ohio

SLACK Incorporated, 6900 Grove Road, Thorofare, NJ 08086-9447

Publisher: John H. Bond
Acquisitions Editor: Amy E. Drummond
Associate Editor: Jennifer J. Cahill
Art Director: Linda Baker

Many of these essays originally appeared in "From Dorko's Desk," a column run regularly in PT Forum from March 1990 to June 1995.

Dorko, Barrett L.
    Shallow dive: essays on the craft of manual care/Barrett L. Dorko.
        p. cm.
    Includes bibliographical references.
    ISBN 1-55642-294-6
    1. Physical therapy. I. Title.
    [DNLM: 1. Physical Therapy—personal narratives. WB 460 D6995s 1995]
RM705.D67 1995
615.8'2—dc20
DNLM/DLC
for Library of Congress

                                                                    95-37787

Printed in the United States of America

Published by: SLACK Incorporated
             6900 Grove Road
             Thorofare, NJ 08086-9447 USA
             Telephone: 609-848-1000
             Fax: 609-853-5991

Contact SLACK Incorporated for more information about other books in this field or about the availability of our books from distributors outside the United States.

Last digit is print number: 10 9 8 7 6 5 4 3 2 1

DEDICATION

This book is dedicated to my parents,
Margaret Elizabeth Hinske Dorko and Andrew John Dorko, Sr.
They taught me how to read, how to write,
and how to open my heart.

CONTENTS

SECTION III:
TELLING THE TALE 74

SECTION V:
FOCUSING ON THE THERAPIST

INTRODUCTION

SHALLOW DIVE

When I was about 8 years old, my parents bought an above-ground pool. Back then this consisted entirely of a circular wire fence and a big piece of blue plastic draped within and filled with water.

Our pool was just over 3 feet deep and maybe 8 feet across. Today, this is exactly how far I can swim before I start to flail and sink.

My father pulled a picnic bench over next to the pool and we started diving in. I don't mean we jumped, we went headfirst.

Dad said we should "shallow dive" and as he said this would always sweep his hand, palm down, across his chest as if it were skipping lightly off of something I couldn't see. I got the idea.

This image of the pool and my father keeps floating through my head these days and I even began a workshop with the story recently in hopes of seeing where it might lead. I am convinced that when the unconscious brings something forth persistently in this way that a fuller expression of it will reveal a meaning relevant and helpful for our current lives.

As I write this I am attending a national convention of the American Physical Therapy Association. Each year I attend this and similar meetings in order to market my workshops, perhaps learn something relevant to my clinical work, and, I suppose, network with my colleagues. I hesitate to use that last description because I can't help but feel that my relationship to my own profession is more accurately described as a web and not a net. That is to say I feel attached but not especially safe. My choice to remain in the profession helps me to remain connected to scientific principles that I find comforting, but at times the language of research and the tendency to focus on tiny parts of human anatomy or function bewilder me. I wonder if I missed a major portion of my training and I often feel I have to hide my enormous lack of knowledge, knowledge of things that seem so important to others.

I live at the edges of these meetings, sitting in the back of every lecture so that I might make an easy, unobtrusive exit. Any time I hear the speaker use a work like "prostaglandin" I can feel myself begin to move irresistibly toward the door. I belong to no committees or task forces. I sit quietly during the many political discussions and wander around alone much of the day. Sometimes I resemble a hockey player who has lost track of the puck.

I have the impression that many in therapy, especially in the manual end of it, feel a persistent frustration born of the fact that although we are supposed to change various organs within a patient's interior, our direct mechanical effect stops pretty much at the surface. Beneath the skin are many processes and bits of anatomy we would love to grip. We aren't allowed to literally do this and so we have developed many elaborate means of affecting change with devices other than our hands. I will admit I don't know much about that form of care.

Whatever I might say about the profound effect manual care might potentially have, it still begins on the surface, and what I do mechanically ends there as well. Like my peripheral presence at these conferences, I move forward headfirst but I remain shallow. I don't dive deep into the politics or administrative intricacies of my profession, but I don't think I'm entirely in the dark. It occurs to me that on the surface of any body of water you can see a lot that can't be seen in the depths.

What I love, what I want to be good at, am good at, isn't taught at national meetings. It is learned in solitary moments with patients, while reading journals and books, some of them obscure and seemingly unrelated to therapy. And, for me, while writing about it as truthfully as I can.

I'm still diving shallow, and the nature of my work will permit nothing more. But I feel that this approach has been sufficient to practice manual care effectively, and, in the end, enough to help me see that the important diving I do is not outward, but within myself.

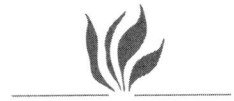

INTRODUCTION

THE CRAFT OF MANUAL CARE

In Old English, the word "craeft" meant "strength or courage." In modern usage, "craft" became synonymous with expertness, skill, or mastery. I also read that craft might be used to connote trickery or deceitfulness.

The distinctions between craft and art are not precise, and it seems that often it is left up to the one viewing an object or a performance whether what they see is one or the other.

I am drawn to calling what I've done for many years with my voice, my hands, and my presence a craft for reasons that feel right though I might not be able to explain them entirely. I understand that some in the community of art tend to distinguish art as more two dimensional, and craft in three dimensions, and that sounds like body work to me. I like the reference to trickery found in the obscure definitions of the word because much of what I do is difficult to see and often produces surprises.

But most of all I like the old references to strength and courage from which the word originally arises.

Today we live in a world where actually touching another person who is not in some way intimately related to you, or who is not passing through some relationship of commerce or perfunctory social discourse, is quite uncommon. It is certainly not expected. I could walk the crowded streets of a large city, eat at a busy diner, ride the buses, check into a hotel, attend a concert, all without once feeling another's hand unless it were passing me something and it were not possible to let the item intervene. This is usually possible.

Those of us who have chosen to enter a kind of work that not only requires that we touch others, but touch them in a way that they cannot ignore, are doing something that requires courage. Doing this, we must remain steady in our resolve to remain present with the changes that inevitably occur, and this requires an endurance and intellectual strength only study and some passion for the work itself can supply.

I am fearful though of making too much of the therapist's skill. I think that it often has been raised to a degree that blinds us to something no real craftsman would ignore: the materials.

Sometimes I'll ask a group of therapists the following question: If I were to point at a wall and ask you to make a hole in it, what would be the first thing you would like to know?

I can't imagine any craftsman not wanting to know first of all what the wall was made of. Only after this was known would they choose the tool or force necessary and no more. I find that many therapists only want to know what size the hole should be, and that says a lot about the current state of manual care.

As much as anything else, these essays are about the materials we have chosen to work with, and I can't imagine anything more or less likely to change, more potentially volatile, less predictable, or more likely to change those who touch it than the human body.

These essays are about what it is like to spend each day with the task of manual caring and what might happen if we attended to the stories we heard and told ourselves. They are about the peripheral issues of anatomy, physiology, emotion, failure, success, and being the imperfect human each of us is.

They all begin with what I have come to know as a craft. I expect to improve my skill and knowledge the rest of my life if only I can sustain the courage and strength it requires.

I hope that from these essays others will learn that somehow without blades, hammers, or anesthesia, profound changes in humans can occur, and that painful technique is largely unnecessary.

I believe this is true because the materials of my craft have shown me this again and again. The answers are in the patients, and they are the ones who have inspired this book.

SECTION I

MAKING SENSE

While speaking to a class about patients with prolonged and bizarre symptoms that have proved unresponsive to traditional means of care, a highly respected clinician and researcher recently mentioned my name. "You know," he said, "these people make sense to Barrett."

I heard of this the next day and spent a while trying to figure out whether or not it was a compliment. I decided that it was.

It seems that I have spent most of my time in the clinic as an interpreter and translator. In fact, I know that people "make sense" to me only when I understand how what they say might be explained in another way. When the underlying processes that produce symptoms are not obvious, special knowledge is required to explain the patient's feeling of change. It has been my experience that the sources of that knowledge might range far beyond what a physical therapist might be expected to study. But does it matter that I wasn't taught how to understand my patients while in school? I have yet to meet a patient that wasn't primarily interested in what I knew today, not what I learned, or managed not to learn, 20 years ago.

In an effort to make sense out of what I hear and see and feel in my patients, I have had to relinquish some cherished ideas about the posture, structure, and changeable nature of the body. This doesn't bother me, although I know many wonderful therapists who will hang on to time-honored notions despite all evidence to the contrary. This attitude isn't new. In fact, Tolstoy described the situation this way in the latter part of the 19th century:

"I know that most men, including those at ease with problems of the greatest complexity, can seldom accept even the simplest and most obvious truth if it be such as would oblige them to admit the falsity of conclusions which they have delighted in explaining to colleagues, which they have proudly taught to others, and which they have woven, thread by thread, into the fabric of their lives."

Tolstoy's remarkable insights into the nature of chronic pain are evident in his short story "The Death of Ivan Illych," which inspired my essay "Nothing's Changed."

If I do indeed have the ability to make sense of the symptoms my patients report and translate them into images to which we can all relate, I think it's because I have always been willing to accept the premise that many things may have multiple meanings. I am ready to admit that the reasons people become impaired and pain ridden are usually not simple or singular, and that recovery might be equally mysterious and unpredictable. I think it's absolutely essential that we do not at the same time accept explanations that violate physical law or require bodily tissue to do things we know that it cannot do.

Since what I actually do clinically is often considered "alternative care," I walk a fine line in an effort to make sense to my patients and my colleagues.

In this section, I have included essays that reflect our knowledge of biophysics, neurobiology, cellular mechanics related to touch, reflexive reactions, and fractal geometry. I draw conclusions but don't often state opinions. I stick to facts whenever they are known and relate clinical phenomena to research.

Despite my personal inclination toward classic literature, I feel an obligation as a physical therapist to explain what I see in the clinic in a scientifically acceptable way. I'm certainly quick to criticize others when they ignore physical law and current literature (see "The Relativity of Wrong," "Connecting the Hemispheres," and "Ockham's Razor").

It also seems evident to me that science teaches us that there is a great deal we will never be able to know or predict with certainty. This is the main idea behind "The Shapes Within."

Although many in therapy pursue the algorithms, protocols, and predictable responses we expect research to provide, I find that it often tells us to go back and find a more reasonable interpretation of what we thought we saw. And then do it again.

In 1992 I was an invited speaker at the national convention of The American Physical Therapy Association. The topic was cranial technique and the theory behind its application and effect. Early in my talk, I cited recently published articles on "facilitated communication" that had appeared in Clinical Management, *a publication sponsored by my professional association.*

The article described the remarkable success a technique of gentle handling had on an autistic child, enabling him to communicate for the first time his specific thoughts, feelings, desires, and love for his mother.

I had read of similar claims with this technique by the originator of facilitated communication in Australia and her students and advocates now in the United States. I had read that in some cases these children no longer needed actual contact on their hands by another as they manually indicated or typed out their messages. In some cases, it was claimed that they needn't be touched at all.

I believed it. After all, this information was being disseminated by authorities in my own profession, and I assumed that they knew that extraordinary claims required extraordinary evidence and that they had this in hand.

I also liked what the articles said about approaching others with some confidence in their skills and intelligence because I try to do that in my own practice.

I was wrong.

Since that time, facilitated communication as a reliable technique has been entirely discredited. It seems that what was being seen was nothing more than the unconscious expression of the facilitator, not the child. The child had become the planchette of a Ouija board and, once again, the shadow of the clinician came forward because we had not adequately acknowledged its presence. The desire to believe that these children could be reached in a simple way, that they were normally intelligent, and that they could tell us they loved their mothers clouded our objectivity and scientific sensibilities.

I am on record at that conference believing what I had read, and proposing my work was similarly effective.

I was wrong and I am perfectly willing to admit it.

It will happen again.

Selected Reading
I'm not handicapped in my brain. *Clinical Management*.1992;12(3).

THE RELATIVITY OF WRONG

In an old episode of "Saturday Night Live," Steve Martin plays a medieval barber. Jane Curtin brings to him her obviously ill daughter (Laraine Newman) for treatment. Martin looks at her and says, "Don't worry good woman, we used to think that something like this was caused by a witch's curse or the ingestion of some devilish vapors. (He stifles a laugh.) But now we know that it is actually due to a small toad or dwarf lying in her stomach."

Thus we witness the progress of science.

Lewis Thomas likens the footing that scientific research and knowledge provides us to an unsteady, shifting mass. He states, "Human knowledge doesn't stay put, it evolves by what we call trial and error, or, as is more usually the sequence, error and trial."

Making progress on a shifting mass would be near to impossible if no firm footholds ever appeared. Several physical laws first described by Newton provided the stability that our quest for knowledge required to move ahead and were a death knell for alchemy and medieval barbers.

Milton Rothman, a physicist, feels that we can use our knowledge of physical law not only to make educated judgments about the plausibility of some of the claims of research, but also to decide what may not occur, no matter how it might appear. He likens such statements as, "Nothing is known for sure" and "Nothing is impossible" to myths, maintained through the force of their psychological power. He points out that the law of conservation of energy has not only stood the test of our time but that through our measurement of starlight, it has been true for millions of years within the space of the observable universe. This makes perpetual motion machinery and the mainstays of parapsychology (precognition, ESP, dowsing, etc.) difficult to accept.

We can view our progress in physical therapy as dependent upon our grasp of physical law and work to explain clinical phenomena within its boundaries. Without this firm footing we run the risk of sliding back toward medieval lunacy.

There's one more issue here. The frightening frequency with which treatment protocols have changed in the past two decades.

One gets the feeling that at the very least our previous care was inadequate if not actually wrong for the problem. However, we must understand that our current knowledge of disease and dysfunction is a consequence of the latest scientifically deduced paradigm. We know that such knowledge has always progressed from the relatively less correct to the more correct model. This is usually the end result of more accurate measuring devices. The introduction of computerized and highly sensitive sensors that reveal the patient's activity is far more likely to change our method of management than the discovery of some previously unknown anatomy.

We have been relatively wrong in the past, and sometime in the future today's method of care will be considered inadequate. As long as our techniques depend upon well-known physical law we will progress with sure footing and we will be able to look back without stifling a laugh.

Selected Reading

Rothman M. Myths about science...and belief in the paranormal. *Skeptical Inquirer.* 1989;Fall.

Thomas L. On the uncertainty of science. *Harvard Magazine.* 1980;Sept/Oct.

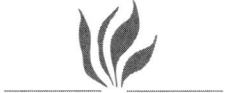

CONNECTING THE HEMISPHERES

The subject of hemispheric specialization has gotten a real workout in both the scientific community and in the popular media during the past 20 years. When Ornstein published the *Psychology of Consciousness* in 1970, he proposed that much of Western society was guilty of overusing the left half of their brains, thus producing a technological and strictly rational culture as opposed to the intuitive, mystical East.

Beyond the verbal/nonverbal distinction that had long been accepted, he proposed that the hemispheres represented alternate ways of knowing. Many others have expanded upon this and have suggested that there are many more distinctions characterizing the two sides of our brain. This seems to have evolved into a kind of "dichotomania" that proposes that our hemispheres process information in opposing ways, for example, rational/metaphoric, intellectual/intuitive, realistic/impulsive, or historical/timeless, to name a few. I personally wonder how much of this is pure speculation and whether many of these terms are not actually separate or distinct qualities, but just extremes of a set of continuous behaviors.

It was also recently proposed that touch elicits emotional response and is therefore a right brain function. "Touch shifts functioning to right brain dominance, [allowing] a direct communication with the right brain."

Oh? There are many ways of touching another. The spectrum runs from an infant's grasp to the kind of thing we see Mike Tyson do on HBO. When it is suggested that hemispheric dominance may be manipulated with the touch of another I begin to wonder about how that has been determined. I suspect that it is an attempt to use some pop-psychology to explain clinical phenomena. Of course, I might just be too "left-brained" to gather all of that. People like me have difficulty seeing things in the intuitive, holistic, and cosmically significant way that the creative sorts in therapy do.

In order to add some fuel to the fire, I'd like to point out that some suggest that strictly separating the functions and expressions of the hemispheres is full of problems. Sacks feels that the hemispheres are merely suited for different dimensions and stages of processing. He reminds us that while the right brain is more active during novel or unexpected situations, the left brain becomes dominant once the situation has been "decoded." This shift is concurrent with the acquisition of skill. "Naive ears hear music on the right [but] experts hear it on the left" and "It is true that all who acquire skill [at] all the higher reaches of scientific or artistic intelligence require representational systems that are functionally similar to language; all of them seem to move to becoming left hemisphere skills."

It appears that the real experts in any endeavor, no matter how artistic it may be considered, are actually using their left brain when they are really in the know. I see a movie with my right brain, Siskel and Ebert with their left.

The hemispheres needn't be at odds. Sagan writes soothingly of this controversial subject: "The search for patterns (right brain) without critical analysis (left brain), and rigid skepticism (left again) without a search for patterns (right, of course), are the antipodes of incomplete science. To solve complex problems requires both hemispheres: the path to the future lies through the corpus callosum. We might say that human culture is the function of the corpus callosum...because every structure in the brain plays a role in human behavior, and human culture is a function of human behavior."

I think I should stop worrying about which half of my head is processing what I see or hear. There doesn't seem to be any fighting over dominance inside me. The fighting is between the people around me.

Selected Reading

Manheim C, Lavett D. *Craniosacral Therapy and Somato-Emotional Release.* Thorofare, NJ: SLACK Inc; 1989:61-62.

Orstein R. *Psychology of Consciousness.* New York, NY: Penguin; 1970.

Sacks O. Seeing Voices, *A Journey Into the World of the Deaf.* Berkeley, Calif: University of California Press; 1989:104-110.

Sagan C. *The Dragons of Eden.* New York, NY: Random House; 1977.

Springer S, Deutsch G. *Left Brain, Right Brain.* New York, NY: Freeman & Co; 1985:237-288.

THE SIGNIFICANCE OF GRAVITY

I read recently of the actual effect of the moon's gravitational pull on the ocean and how it was just one of several factors leading to tidal activity.

The article reinforced the fact that gravitational forces have their most significant effect on extremely large objects and that human beings are much more likely to respond to the changes in electromagnetism that courses through us in the form of nervous depolarization and chemical bonding.

On the other hand, we seem both metaphorically and actually like the ocean in our chemical constituents, internal rhythms, and the fractal geometry of some internal organs as well as the skin. I think all of this lends our bodies their pliable and unpredictable nature.

Quick, what are the four forces in the universe?

I love this question. I memorized the answer some time ago and it's one of those things that can make you appear rather smart. I've always needed things like that. Of course, I sometimes have difficulty getting this question into dinner conversations or light chatter with wine and hors d'oeuvres. Nevertheless, I know the answer and I would hate to keep this information to myself. The answer is gravity, electromagnetism, and the weak and strong nuclear forces.

It wasn't until recently that I began to wonder if this knowledge held any significance for me. I guess it must have been my exposure to the nontraditional forms of therapy that made me think about the physics of energy transference and what the laws governing this can allow us to presume.

I had been under the impression that gravity was my main concern as a therapist trying to alter the movement of others. The effect of this force is so pervasive that I always felt at odds with it. I came across some interesting work that has made me think again, however, and it has altered my perception a bit.

Sheldon Glashow explains the functions of the known forces in a way I'd not seen before. He points out that the effect that a force has on an object depends upon the size of the object itself. The stars and planets, the oceans and continents are moved predominantly by gravity. Of the forces, this is by far the weakest, but it makes up for that by the sheer number of atoms exerting this force continuously and in only one direction.

Everything smaller than a major land mass and larger than an atom is primarily affected by electromagnetism. The supremacy of this force is evident every time we get out of a chair. Gravity tries, but it must give way to the vastly superior strength that chemical reactions (an expression of electromagnetism) can generate. Of course, electromagnetism also differs from gravity in that it can act upon any object in two opposing directions at the same time, effectively canceling itself out. Another difference is that it is not capable of exerting its force over the distance gravity is known to.

The nuclear forces govern movement in a realm too small to measure with a goniometer so I don't normally consider them in the clinic.

So what has this got to do with therapy? Well, for a long time I waged a war against this persistent and unfatiguable thing that came up out of the ground and commonly pulled me in a direction that was often inconvenient. I spent a lot of time and money getting "Rolfed." According to the founder of this technique, it was supposed to align me so that gravity "lifted me up." (I never did understand that.) I certainly changed but I'm fairly certain that the gravitational field in Ohio didn't.

Glashow's essay reminded me that while gravity might have been the first force that I observed and was aware of feeling as an infant, my scientific background had altered my feelings with an important fact. The fact is I can generate enough force from within me to overcome the pull of this entire planet. The moon might produce an ocean tide but I can raise water from the Pacific in the opposite direction with my own hand.

As a therapist I must remain mindful of potential falls by my patients. Gravity, essentially a force outside of our control, is always something I must consider. It's nice to remember though that each of us is capable of generating something much stronger. Something that is remarkably controllable and can be enhanced with the help that therapy provides.

Selected Reading
Glashow S. Tangled in supersting. *The Sciences*. 1988;May/Jun.
Quincey P. Why we are unmoved as oceans ebb and flow. *Skeptical Inquirer*. 1994;18(5):509-515.

TSUNAMI

In 1960, there was an earthquake in Chile. Twenty-two hours later, 199 people in Japan had drowned.

The transfer of energy across thousands of miles of open water is accomplished by a waveform known as a soliton. A tidal wave is perhaps the best known and most dramatic expression of this naturally occurring phenomenon, but it is important to understand that you don't need an earthquake to generate energy transference in this way. In the 1830s, Scott Russell, a British engineer, described waves of remarkable longevity in the canals near his home. They were formed by the sudden stopping of a ship with a distinctly shaped bow. It is the closest thing to a perpetual motion machine seen in nature.

Mathematical breakthroughs in the 1960s allowed scientists to recognize the presence of this waveform and its frequent occurrence. We now produce it ourselves and pump light through fiber-optic cables with remarkable efficiency.

Although biological structures are not especially convenient for the study of waveforms, careful observation reveals that solitons are a common form of energy transference in the body. Their presence explains many of the mysteries surrounding energy conversion as well.

When someone is touched, tremors are sent through the medium of the body. The waves created by the mechanical deformation of the tissue usually disperse very rapidly and affect only the inert or contractile tissue immediately adjacent.

The waves of energy that accompany the reflexive effect of handling are quite different. Their potential movement is dependent upon the anatomical relationships of the neurons involved and the nature of the stimulation (i.e., it is inversely proportional to the force of the stimulus). The packets of energy that form the nerve impulse travel as a seismic wave would across the ocean. Unless it runs into an island, the energy necessary for it to continue long distances will remain present.

The combination of gentle touch, facilitated nervous tissue, and an environment conducive to internal awareness commonly produces the report of sensation and pain relief in distant parts. I personally refer to the technique as "simple contact."

It was never my experience that pressing, rubbing, poking, or manipulating another had the same effect.

When I began to see the body as an animated fluid mass, it responded in kind, revealing its tendency toward health as well as its hidden islands of dysfunction.

Now when I touch patients and they tell me of sensation elsewhere, I don't think they are crazy. Instead, I appreciate the powerful movement of energy within.

Suggested Reading
Briggs J, Peat F. *Turbulent Mirror.* New York, NY: Harper and Row; 1989.
Scott A. The solitary wave. *The Sciences.* 1990;Mar/Apr.

SUPERGLUE

Ever get some superglue stuck on your finger? Can you think of anything more irritating that is not in any way painful?

Anyone who thinks that I have some special manual skill because of my years in the profession should watch me use a tube of glue. I have learned to get the glue and nail polish remover out at the same time. The glue on the finger sends a persistent message: "Something is wrong here and I want it fixed now!"

Mechanical deformation of the skin somehow becomes an electrical signal in the brain. The mechanisms responsible for this have come to light only in the past decade and I think they explain much about manual care.

Sensation follows depolarization and this requires the movement of ions across the neuronal membrane. Ions cross the membrane at specific channels that are opened or closed depending upon the chemical or electrical activity locally. This process was confirmed many years ago but did not explain how touch led to ion channel opening in nervous tissue.

In 1984, Sachs and Guharay identified ion channels in cellular tissue aside from the neuron. These opened when sufficient mechanical force was used to deform the cytoskeleton and were called "stretch-activated ion channels." The researchers also found that increased membranous tension of the cell enhanced the effect of deformation (i.e., a tight cell membrane displayed more ion channel opening when deformed).

The mechanism is remarkably similar to that of a canvas tent in a rainstorm. A tent will not allow leakage as long as no puddles form on its surface or no one stretches the canvas by leaning into it. Deforming the canvas orchestrates an opening in the fibers sufficient to allow rain to seep through.

When I touch the epithelial tissue, I similarly orchestrate an opening in the cell wall and an influx of potassium triggers mechanoreceptor depolarization. This is how touch leads to sensation.

By understanding this mechanism, we can appreciate the varieties of response to be had by touching different parts of the body. If cellular tautness is prevalent in an area of pain or scarring, it follows that mechanical stimulation here would have its greatest effect. For me, this solves most of the riddles surrounding trigger points.

Now, back to the superglue. I have the impression that its presence on my finger blocks the initial processes of tactile sensation profoundly. I become suddenly unable to open the ion channels at this spot. Clothing does not do anything more than dampen the process.

When I think about it, I feel a sense of loss. It is akin to a sudden deafness or as if someone has just turned out the lights. It does not hurt, but I really would prefer an immediate return of my normal senses. I learn again that my sensibilities are a gift I appreciate most when they are lost.

Selected Reading

Guharay, Sachs F. Stretch-activated single ion channel currents in tissue-cultured embryonic chick skeletal muscle. *Journal of Physiology.* 1984;352:685-701.

Suggested Reading

Sachs F. The intimate sense: understanding the mechanics of touch. *The Sciences.* 1988;Jan/Feb.

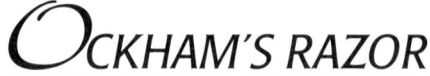

OCKHAM'S RAZOR

"Plurality should not be assumed without necessity."

William of Ockham, 1285-1349

A few weeks ago a patient at her second visit told me she had been warmer the previous few days.

"This boggles my mind because I went through past-life transgression therapy a while ago and found out I had frozen to death. I thought that's why I was always cold."

I thought she was cold because she was sympathetic dominant. After some corrective movement and regular diaphragmatic breathing, her peripheral blood flow had increased. This is the only way anybody ever warms up without becoming feverish.

In the 14th century, theologian and logician William of Ockham argued that phenomena should be explained in the simplest possible way and that we should differentiate between evidence and degrees of probability.

Such thinking has become known as "Ockham's Razor," and as a principle of logic and deduction it is especially useful in medicine.

For example, when a patient is late for an appointment, I might try to explain this in many ways. If I consider the time of day and the traffic patterns between my office and his or her home, the delay might be easily understood and perfectly plausible. Without Ockham's Razor, I might seriously consider that he or she had been abducted by aliens. See what I mean?

Some of the more esoteric forms of manual care might gain acceptance if we used Ockham's severely rational scrutiny to explain their effects.

In a lab in New York, Dimitrios Kostopoulous, MA, PT, works to prove that gentle pressures on the forehead (frontal bone) lead to measurable deformation of the falx cerebri. He has accomplished this, and now we are free to consider the mechanical and reflexive implications of that movement.

It seems so simple a thing—you push on something and something attached to it moves. But the traditions of medicine do not include movement within the dural structures without significant or even dangerous outside forces. Something like a Rocky Marciano left hook.

If the cranial "vault" is indeed just that, any technique that deforms it would be potentially harmful. Florence Kendall states, "If the sagittal suture opened, the patient would split in two!"

But many techniques of bodywork employ gentle forces at the head, and their effects might be simply explained if we consider that movement of the dural and its intimately connected neural tissue took place. Without that mechanism, we are led toward notions of "energy flow," "cranial rhythm," or "body memory" that cannot withstand the scrutiny of the medical community or Ockham's admonition.

Sometimes the therapy community rejects explanations that are new simply because they defy tradition. Sometimes therapists adhere to the status quo out of loyalty to methods that have the weight of time on their side, if not effectiveness or logic.

When we touch each other's heads, the effects are both reflexive and mechanical. The mechanical effects occur in highly innervated tissue, the force required is very small and potentially harmless. These are simple facts that might explain a lot.

I think Ockham would have liked them.

<u>Selected Reading</u>
Kendall F. Catherine Worthingham Fellow Forum; Cincinnati, Ohio; June 1993.
Kostopoulous DC, Keramidas G. Changes in elongation of falx cerebri during craniosacral therapy techniques applied on the skull of an embalmed cadaver. *J Craniomandibular Practice.* 1992;10(1).
Kostopoulous DC, Keramidas G. Changes in magnitude of relative cerebri during the application of external forces on the frontal bone of an embalmed cadaver. *PT Forum.* 1991;10(10).

THERE'S A WEB

There's a web within the body that exists as no other organ. It begins in the brain and extends to the very edge of the epithelium. It doesn't display any breaks, but only a seemingly infinite branching as it embraces, informs, and accepts messages from each cell.

The shape of this organ provides important clues about its internal activity. Its architecture is that of a "fractal." A fractal is a structure that is self-similar across scale: something that appears the same in macro- and microcosm. It is known that these structures are commonly the remnants of chaotic dynamics; activity that displays an order and periodicity only when viewed in a certain way. The waves of the ocean create a fractal coastline.

This organ's presence in the body is expressed in a undulating fashion, evident to the naked eye in its trunks and larger branches and, to the microscope, within its deepest layers and tiniest extension. We know the loss of this naturally occurring slackness has profound and immediate effects on the normal function of the web and, as in any web, mechanical strain in one part is potentially reflected to the whole.

Connective tissue is unlike this web in several important ways. While connective tissue acts as an anchor, a chemical filter, a dividing line, and fluid crystal, it is largely non-living and incredibly variable in its consistency and function. Its architecture is non-fractal, thereby reducing its ability to change rapidly in response to gentle stimuli in any lasting fashion. Its work occurs in slow motion.

The web I speak of isn't just mechanically continuous, its "plumbing" extends without the protection of valves across lengthy extensions of a single cell, perhaps a meter in length. The movement of fluid through the web is dependent upon vascular support that reacts powerfully to compression or tension or endocrine activity. This blood flow can change as quickly as a blush might appear, and a blush might have nothing more than a thought behind its origin.

As you might have guessed already, this organ is also continuously connected in an electrical fashion. Beyond that, it has been demonstrated that the packets of energy flowing through this tissue travel as a tidal wave across the ocean. They lose very little energy over vast distances and the proper stimulation to the web can affect the body from head to toe, though it might be remarkably gentle.

This web functions marvelously most of the time. Its infinite infoldings, the collateral vascular support, the enveloping connective tissue, and its topography all act to protect it.

But when its movement is restricted and its vascular and intracellular flow is diminished, the same widespread presence that enhances its power can lead to symptoms throughout the body, symptoms with an invisible origin and signs difficult to palpate in the usual way. Maybe when we understand the web in all of these ways we can find some path toward it.

Suggested Reading

Goldberger A, et al. Chaos and fractals in human physiology. *Scientific American.* 1990;Feb.

Lipsitz L, et al. Loss of "complexity" in aging potential applications of fractals and chaos theory to senescence. *JAMA.* 267(13).

Scott A. The solitary wave. *The Sciences.* 1990;Mar/Apr.

THE SHAPES WITHIN–I

Hold on to your hats. This essay has been brewing for a couple of years. This means the material is complex and perhaps deeply disturbing to some segment of the PT community. Still, the subject is too compelling to hold in, and the implications of what I am suggesting are large. But these ideas drive my daily practice and that's what I write about here.

I have long felt that the phrase "soft tissue" has been difficult to define. Mainly because I never hear the alternative "hard tissue." Oh, I suppose a case could be made for the idea that bony or periarticular structures are separate from soft tissues in some way, but I've never heard anyone speak passionately or convincingly of this. Without that, soft tissue becomes something like light without darkness. In other words, not possible.

In fact, any step dissection of the body reveals that the deepest layers of fascia are continuous with the periosteum. On a molecular level, these two tissues simply have different concentrations of mineral salts and both are categorized as connective tissue.

How can I move so-called soft tissue and not take the bone with it?

In addition to this vague and (I think) spurious distinction between hard and soft tissue, I have long been struck by the connotations of the statement, "This patient has soft tissue problems." I think the distinct underlying message is, "This patient is never going to fully recover." Or, "I did some soft tissue work." This means: "I applied heavy pressure with my knuckles." (Boy, am I going to get into trouble for saying that.)

So, if I don't think hard and soft tissues are effectively separate in either an anatomical or clinical sense, what kind of distinctions in body tissue are useful?

Let's try this: Look around the room and consider the shapes you see. For the most part, manufactured goods these days contain simple lines, curves, or square corners that are easily described using classic Euclidean formulas. We live in boxes, sit on rectangles, and bathe within ovals.

Now look outside. The shapes occurring in the natural world often defy any effort to accurately calculate the area of their shape. Especially if they are examined carefully.

A common geometric feature of the natural world is self-similarity across scale. That is, a structure's tendency to appear the same when viewed from a variety of distances, like the branching of a tree or a coastline, or a river. Such shapes are called "fractals" and their presence indicates something important about the forces that formed them and the activity within them.

Fractals appear where chaotic, turbulent, unpredictable activity meets stable, linear, dependable forces. Once the characteristics of their shape are understood, their presence all around us becomes evident.

The reason I mention all of this is because this geometry of nature is largely responsible for activity in the body that confounds the therapy and medical communities. My next essay, "The Shapes Within—II", proposes a new categorization of tissue and offers an explanation for the varieties of effect manual care might produce.

<u>Suggested Reading</u>
Dorko BL. *Fractal Geometry and Manual Care.* Available from the author.

THE SHAPES WITHIN–II

In my last essay I proposed that separating the body into soft and hard tissue was not anatomically accurate or clinically useful. What I am suggesting here is that a different classification is valid and clinically important.

The new science of chaos has helped a variety of disciplines see the changes that occur within phenomena in a new way. Where order was thought to rule, randomness became evident and where prediction had been thought impossible, a strict pattern of behavior could be demonstrated.

The aspect of chaos theory that concerns us here is the relation of activity to geometric shape. I wrote last time of "fractals," shapes that branch respectively in their periphery and defy accurate measurement of their surface area.

Where fractal shapes are seen, we know that chaotic, unpredictable activity is occurring adjacent to otherwise stable structures. Where the ocean (driven by the chaos of weather) meets the shore, a fractal coastline is always produced.

In the body, many organs and tissues do not display fractal geometric shape. These include bones and other connective tissues, muscle and tendons. The significance of their linear shape lies in their predictable response to provocation, stimulation, or injury. Where dysfunction or pain arises from these structures, tests of provocation provide clear responses that are easily interpreted. Management of linear tissue problems can follow protocols that everyone agrees upon. I believe sports medicine has refined our knowledge of these tissues to an amazing degree.

But there are tissues that branch like a tree and flow like a river. Disorders affecting such tissues prove far more difficult to control because a variety of factors always contribute to the eventual expression of the tissue's current function. Let me ask:

- How many things might alter blood pressure?
- How difficult is it to predictably reduce hypertension?
- What is the geometric shape of the circulatory system?

I propose that the answers to these questions are always linked. For physical therapists, those problems that involve nervous irritation often are the least likely to follow a predictable path of recovery or respond consistently to a protocol of management. Wildly fluctuating location of pain, unexpected responses to changes in position, pressure, treatment, rest, work, and the circumstances of life are common in spinal pain, headache, carpal tunnel and thoracic outlet syndromes, and sciatica. Controlling these can seem as difficult as altering the course of a river by placing a rock in one of its branches.

Maybe this is why many in our business much prefer the certainty of knee rehabilitation to the treatment of any spinal pain. Without knowing it, we have distinguished between the linear and fractal tissues of the body and chosen the stable ones. Ask yourself, "Does this patient have a disorder of the linear or fractal structures within their bodies?" The answer and its implications alter every aspect of the clinical picture and our philosophy of care.

In fact, the only organ directly accessible to touch, the skin, is a fractal. The next time you touch someone and get an unexpected response, think of that.

SECTION II

ASSESSMENT

Although it would be nice if it were otherwise, the body seems to defy our desire to examine it simply, reliably, consistently, and accurately. There is not a great deal of evidence that visual inspection of the surface will reveal relevant internal processes and in fact we can never be certain that patients, being animated, won't effectively hide their true nature simply because of the situation present in the examining booth. Additionally, we have problems simply seeing and interpreting anything before us.

Techniques of manual and visual examination also present us with the problems of subtlety, ambiguity, and the constantly changing nature of patients in response to the simple act of touch. I'm convinced that our techniques of assessment are primarily affected by the model of the body that we live with. My own model tends to change as the years go by.

CONCRETE

"I really like all the stuff you present, but I work with people who are real left-brained and they need to be able to measure or at least see what's going on before they'll believe anything."

I hear this comment at least once at every workshop. It occurs to me first of all that I am much the same. I like the clear evidence that good research provides clinicians and my articles and lectures are full of excellent references that support my thinking and my approach to patients. But it is evident to me that many therapists would rather I remained the purely intuitive, mystic sort commonly associated with alternative approaches to care. How could I possibly be a member of the lunatic fringe and still read the *APTA Journal*?

Perhaps the essential difference between approaches lies in our model of the body. After all, how we interpret signs or symptoms depends on what we think might cause them. Many of my patients have been previously treated by someone especially interested in their "trigger points." These tender spots on the surface have been prodded, injected, lasered, needled, frozen, elbowed, heated, electrically stimulated, or stretched. Despite all this attention, the trigger points commonly remain or return rapidly. I am willing to concede that some people do get some relief with such treatment.

Irvin Korr wrote of trigger points in 1955, "...something discrete and palpable...something upon which one can place his hand." He emphatically states that to equate this tender spot with the patient's problem is "dangerous and misleading," that to do so is as wrong as identifying glucosuria and not bothering to attend to the underlying diabetes.

Why have we ignored this warning for so many years? Why do we interpret the palpable, local, superficial changes at the surface as something wrong that must be eliminated? Well, it is certainly easier than considering the internal processes that cannot be seen or coerced into submission while in our office. The "left-brained" therapists want something to see so that they can control it. I once worked with a physician who would place a needle into a painful area and move it around: "Does it hurt here...here...here...here?"

If my model of the body were of something that displayed itself with clarity and consistency, trigger points would be a welcomed sight. I would assume that since they weren't ordinarily present, that getting rid of them would somehow be good. If I needed something to measure and see before I began treatment, I would be satisfied.

But the body is not always clear and precise in its appearance. Two things seem to be simultaneously true: the body hides what it needs most deeply to express and it clearly expresses what it most desperately wishes to hide. If that sounds impossible or ambiguous, well, welcome to clinical reality.

I feel that the body is properly described as a metaphor. On its surface and in its expressions or gestures are symbols of inner processes that are sometimes understandable and sometimes mysterious. It would be nice if that which was palpable and measurable consistently represented known lesions or clearly understood dysfunction, but it doesn't.

Sometimes we "concretize" metaphors in order to make them simpler, accessible to everyone and easier to interpret. The human body is not concrete and I can hardly apologize for not teaching as if it were. Actually, I prefer the puzzle. It makes my day much more interesting.

Selected Reading
Korr I. Symposium on the functional implications of segmental facilitation. *JOAO.* 1955;54(5).

Suggested Reading
Dorko B. Palpatory diagnoses and the irritative nerve lesion. *PT Forum.* 1989;8(13).

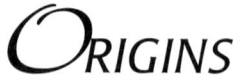ORIGINS

*Origin: The source from which anything arises;
the first stage of existence.
Cause: A thing that exists in such a way that
some specific thing happens as a result.*

Random House College Dictionary

I often ask patients what their previous therapists thought was wrong with them. Commonly they have no idea.

Of course, this is not necessarily the therapist's fault. I'm pretty sure that the same question has been asked of my former patients with the same result. I know I told them.

I begin my workshops with a quote from the neurologist Barry Wyke: "Pain is a disordered affective state brought into being by chemical or mechanical changes in various tissues..." I go on to emphasize that the origins of pain are just two in number: chemical irritation or mechanical deformation. For years I've watched therapists write this down carefully and I know that for most it is new information.

Often I've wondered why this isn't common knowledge and finally I think it's this: As a profession we have concentrated on causes rather than origins. In other words, we have focused on states of function rather than states of being. The former is visible, easier to measure and to push into the desired direction than the latter. States of being involve the whole patient, are less predictable, and require more subjective information than we might ordinarily trust.

Our fixation on function has led to a vast array of techniques that address some cause for the patient's complaint. The patient is moving "wrong," they have poor posture, weak muscles, or shortened connective tissue. They are obese, lack awareness or motivation. Their joints are hypomobile or hypermobile or (if none of this is obvious) they have "microtrauma."

This kind of thinking logically precedes our efforts to treat others as if the origin of pain (usually mechanical deformation) was less important than what the therapist thinks is the cause. Unfortunately, causes have a variable, faddish quality and are strongly influenced by the latest craze in technique.

A return to the origins of pain would make us question the logic of some currently popular causes for pain, and it would certainly explain why many treatments have little or no effect.

If what you are doing does not lead directly to a reduction of the mechanical deformation or chemical irritation in the patient, it probably won't help. When my patients ask me why they hurt, I always return to the origins of pain to explain, and they usually understand and can repeat this to others.

As a physical therapist, my primary concern is with which movements are beneficial, and I search for those.

Suggested Reading

Jayson MI, ed. *The Lumbar Spine and Back Pain*. 4th ed. New York, NY: Churchill Livingstone; 1992.

What's in a Name?

"The physician should speak of that which is invisible. What is visible should belong to his knowledge, and he should recognize illnesses, just as anyone who is not a physician can recognize them from their symptoms. But this is far from making him a physician; he becomes a physician only when he knows that which is unnamed, invisible, and immaterial, yet has its effect."

Paracelsus, German physician/mystic, 1493-1541

There is a trilogy by the fantasy/science fiction writer Ursula K. LeGuin that I read for the first time 20 years ago and continue to return to today. In the land envisioned by LeGuin, everything, including the people, have two names: a "use" name and a "true" name. If you know the true name of an object or a person you have power over them. Those who know all the true names are the wizards of this world.

Eight years ago I was struggling to understand the diagnosis of "fibrositis," so common from one of my referral sources, when I came across an article by the rheumatologist Robert Bennett. After explaining that there is no evidence of inflamed fibers, he defends the diagnosis by evoking the doctrine of nominalism, that illness may be named without it being understood. This naming will suffice until the essential lesion is discovered. Bennett uses lupus as a classic example of nominalistic diagnosis.

Since reading this I have found that most physicians and therapists do not understand the distinction between nominal and essential diagnoses. This causes much confusion in the world of orthopedics where what is wrong is supposed to be visible, or at least palpable.

For several years I have been convinced that the essential lesion my patients suffer from is adverse mechanical tension in the nervous tissue. It is variously named fibrositis, myositis, fibromyalgia, myofibralgia, and probably a few other things outside of Ohio. It doesn't matter. As in LeGuin's fantasy, these are just "use" names, not true ones. Until the essential lesion is identified, our power over it will remain limited. Once we call illness by the name that truly describes it, we become wizards and movement toward health may proceed. Or, at least we know which incantations to use.

Right now the best reference available on tension in the nerves and how to identify its place in many syndromes is *Mobilisation of the Nervous System* by David Butler. I couldn't recommend it more highly.

In LeGuin's fantasy, a young wizard dares to call forth a nameless shadow from beneath the earth. It escapes and cannot be controlled because it has no name. After many trials the wizard embraces the shadow and calls it by his own name, and the danger is past.

I think there may be another essay in that story.

Selected Reading

Bennett R. Does fibrositis exist and can it be treated? *Journal of Musculoskeletal Medicine.* 1984;1(7).

Butler D. *Mobilisation of the Nervous System.* Melbourne: Churchill Livingstone; 1991.

LeGuin UK. *The Earthsea Trilogy.* New York, NY: Bantam; 1968.

$\mathcal{J}$ CAN'T SEE

Darth Vader: "Help me take this mask off."
Luke: "But you'll die."
*Darth Vader: "Nothing can stop that now. Just once, let me look on
you with my own eyes."*

From the final scenes of "Return of the Jedi."

I had the opportunity to go to the top of a mountain in Vail, Colorado last month. It was a cool, clear evening, and a large group of us gathered at the highest point and looked out on a vista that was not only beautiful, it was very different than the land around Cuyahoga Falls, Ohio.

I looked for a few brief moments. Then I found myself doing something very familiar: I stop looking out and I start looking down. I might examine my hands, my shoes, the grass beneath me. While others in the same spot stare enthralled by the view, I find it difficult to stop. I take in what I can quickly see and then withdraw my eyes.

Although well corrected with lenses, I am remarkably nearsighted. I was 7 years old before I knew what normal vision could be like and the moment glasses were placed on my nose remains vivid.

Two years ago I was sent the introduction to a master's thesis by Mari Naumovski, a bodyworker in Canada, entitled "Behind the Eyes: The Speaking of Myopia." Mari writes passionately of her experience of seeing the world through lenses and alternately spending time in the "place of vagueness" that her own eyes can see. Although this place always exists, she spends most of her life covering it with lenses immediately upon waking. I could say the same.

Two weeks after the mountain top in Vail I sat in Denver listening to a Rolfer at the APTA convention. He spoke of how 50% of his training consisted of learning to see postural aberrations and asymmetries in the body before they are palpated and altered with manual care.

I thought of how frustrating looking for subtle changes in body symmetry has always been for me. I still don't visually examine people in anything more than the most superficial way. I've even written of the problems inherent to seeing rounded forms, and I once made a speech about how thinking that you see something influences what the object feels like subsequently. It is called "visual capture" in the literature on perception and it's another reason I've found not to look and invest much in what I see.

Naumovski points out that seeing is more than the ability to access reflected light; it is also a sensual experience. Somewhere behind my eyes I don't process things in the usual way. I lack some kind of sensing that most others have, the ones who linger at the top of a mountain while I look for someone to talk to, something to read.

Having my vision corrected was a wonderful thing, but I have begun to wonder about what I might have learned during the first 7 years of my life. Perhaps I found my other senses more reliable. Maybe some critical early learning that connects sight and sensation was not available to me and my learning style was imprinted in a way that led to a manual strategy of examination and treatment today.

When I think about it, the only time I purposely remove my lenses to see something is once each year at Christmas when I view the tree late at night. If you think there is no gift in myopia, you haven't seen colored lights in this way.

Darth Vader didn't ask for the removal of his helmet. He called it a mask. He understood that lenses not only reveal the world, but hide something as well. In a profession so dependent upon perception, this is something worth considering.

Selected Reading
Dorko BL. *The vision thing*.
Naumovski M. *Behind the eyes: the speaking of myopia*. Master's thesis.

SLOW MOTION

In the moving "Awakenings," Robin Williams delivers a line that lit up something in my head. He asks, "Would a Parkinsonian tremor taken to its furthest extreme produce no tremor at all?" He was referring to the stone-like rigidity of patients who had suffered from a specific form of encephalitis decades before.

Williams portrays a neurologist confronted with a population of patients with whom he was unable to communicate in the usual manner. Inspired by the actual experiences of Oliver Sacks, MD, *Awakenings* deals with Sacks's realization that his seemingly psychotic patients had been rendered akinetic and aphonic by a chemical aberration that could be relieved by doses of L-Dopa.

I read *Awakenings* many years ago, and have been quoting it to my classes since. Although you might imagine that the effect of the medication would form the bulk of this book, it doesn't.

The vast majority of Sacks's writing concerns his minute observation of his patients prior to his administration of the drug. Over and over again he finds, in what appear to be inert beings, indications of normal human emotion and activity. The subtle cues that lead him to the conclusion that his patients are caged physically and not mentally by their disease are obvious only when Sacks takes the time to watch. For hours, days, and weeks he sits silently with his charges and uses a "phenomenological openness" that allows him to see what they do in solitude, quietly, and most of all, slowly.

Our common experience watching the NFL would lead us to believe that viewing events in slow motion would make them easier to see. In fact, something that happens slowly and insidiously can escape our notice completely unless we are persistently vigilant. This is not only true of illness, but the powers of health as well.

If testing is designed to reveal only deficient functioning and if the patient's abilities emerge slowly and quietly, much of what is right with them will be missed.

The movements that Sacks discovered in his patients were not just slow and subdued, they were usually spontaneous as well. Ten years later in *A Leg To Stand On,* Sacks wrote of his prolonged recovery from a knee injury. Although this would ordinarily be considered an "orthopedic" problem, Sacks begins to realize that his problems with sensory agnosia are common among his fellow patients. Almost without exception his physicians are disinterested or disbelieving when he tries to enlist their help.

Beyond that, his recovery is dependent upon movement that is unplanned and improvisational. His formal exercises offer him little more than did traditional testing. As with the "neurologic" patients of his past, his "orthopedic" problems needed time to display the slow motion recovery of coordination that no traditional testing could reveal.

When Robin Williams spoke that line I was reminded of the careful, quiet observation that led to such a notion. That part of our practice lacks drama and pizzazz, but nothing can replace it.

Selected Reading
Sacks O. *A Leg to Stand On*. New York, NY: Summit Books; 1984.
Sacks O. *Awakenings*. New York, NY: EP Dutton; 1974.

ARISTOTLE IN THE CLINIC

"It is the mark of an educated mind to rest satisfied with the degree of precision that the nature of the subject admits, and not to seek exactness when only an approximation is possible."

Aristotle, from "Nicomachean Ethics," Third Century, BC

Sometimes when I read a piece of research in the physical therapy literature, I feel something akin to despair. I am reminded not only of how little I know, but also how much careful work is required to really know anything with certainty. Aristotle's quote is comforting to a degree, but we must remember that he did not write for any refereed journals. In this way, he and I are the same.

I have read and reread an article by Gail M. Jensen, PhD, PT, entitled "Qualitative Methods in Physical Therapy Research: A Form of Disciplined Inquiry" many times and continue to be impressed with its clarity, breadth, and significance to my clinical practice.

Dr. Jensen details the characteristics of various methodologies in qualitative research and contrasts these to more well-known natural science or quantitative approaches. While I cannot describe the entire article, the table of general characteristics within quantitative and qualitative modes of inquiry strikes me as remarkably descriptive of the kind of thinking I most often employ in the clinic.

The dimensions within these two modes of inquiry include the familiar issues of philosophical base, purpose, design, and reality. The quantitative and qualitative modes differ markedly in their approaches to each dimension. Where the former is represented by positivist philosophy that seeks to verify and reduce phenomena to a single reality, the latter is a phenomenological view that discovers and expands what is seen and understood, even proposing multiple realities. I especially like this multiple realities part. Jensen points out that the focus of such research is on the understanding of human behavior from an "insider's perspective." This is identical to the somatic philosophy espoused by Thomas Hanna that I feel is an essential part of all physical therapy practice. It appears that qualitative research requires an accurate description of the patient's experience. They must indicate in some authentic way how it is to be the way they are and how therapeutic intervention alters that. I would imagine that any patient participating in this kind of study would have to see the relevance of the work to his or her condition and its resolution. Such a realization must enhance the validity of the study in a number of ways.

Jensen also emphasizes that in a qualitative mode of inquiry the researcher is the instrument, and that direct personal contact with people is essential. Any clinician who feels that his or her involvement with patients beyond the boundaries of diagnosis precludes the cold, objective view necessary for hard science must be heartened by this. In such research, rich description, long-term participation, and interpretation of subject-generated processes do not cloud our conclusions, but rather lead to more discovery.

There is an elusive quality to people that often spells the difference between success and failure in the clinic. I often wonder if traditional research has any connection to what I do each day. Perhaps in the quality of our patients and the multiple realities revealed through a thoughtful but less rigid approach, I can despair less often and occasionally express what I know to be true.

Selected Reading

Jensen GM. Qualitative methods in physical therapy research: a form of disciplined injury. *Physical Therapy*. 1989;69(6).

THE STATE OF NORTH DAKOTA

"The most critical effect, clinically, of manipulation is the reduction of sympathetic hyperactivity and its pathogenic pain-producing influences."

Irvin Korr

I've seen more wrist splints the past 5 years than in the previous 15. Most of them have been on grocery store checkout clerks.

It would be easy to write of the biomechanics of the wrist and how the repetitive use of a scanner might compromise the median nerve. It's been done.

Ergonomics studies the interface of the work station with the body. As an evolving science it has explained many complaints of pain and prevented or alleviated problems when employed in a timely fashion.

I'm no expert on ergonomics, but as I read of it I begin to think of another interface: that place where the inner life and the outer life of the worker meet. I think this is somewhere beneath the skin.

I always ask my patients if they are commonly chilly or intolerant of a cool breeze. Their response is so often positive that I've come to feel that the internal temperature of the body has a profound impact on whether or not it hurts. Of course, this comes as no great revelation to those who correlate stress to pain. An increase in sympathetic tone with its sweat gland activity and decreased blood flow to the periphery is guaranteed to create a clammy surface that freezes in the wind.

My patients often have the consistency of refrigerated gelatin. They have difficulty changing their shape. This is an expression of a general increase in muscle tone that must accompany their autonomic imbalance. It is called ergotropy, a tendency to work.

I tell them that I want therapy to produce something like the competitive swimmer's body as it approaches the blocks. In this you see fluidity, laxity, and the easy conformity to repetitive movement that lets them swim. Their gelatin is on the stove.

This display of internal warmth is not something I ever see walking into my office for an initial visit. Grocery clerks wearing wrist splints don't look much like this either. They often have a bulky sweater over their uniform while their symptom-free colleagues are comfortable without one.

The mechanics of a job are important to consider. But I wonder if we emphasize enough the adaptive potential of the person being asked to do it. This is different then flexibility and changes rapidly in response to stress, position, and movement. It can change as quickly as a thought.

Explaining physiologic states to a grocery clerk can be challenging. I tell them that on the inside they're in the "state" of North Dakota. They need to move south. Alabama would be nice.

Irvin Korr started observing the effects of manual care in 1953. Twenty-five years later he certainly knew what it had to accomplish in order to help. It had to warm people up from the inside-out. He understood that pain is often the result of a subtle process, not an obvious event. Until we attend to that process, the people who make wrist splints and sweaters will do pretty well.

Selected Reading

Dorko BL. Adaptive potential: a new concept in pain of mechanical origin. *PT Forum.* 1988;7(29).

Korr I. *The Neurobiologic Mechanisms in Manipulative Therapy.* New York, NY: Plenum Press; 1978.

THE VIEW FROM INSIDE

In his 1981 Nobel lecture, psychobiologist Roger W. Sperry spoke of his research into the nature of consciousness and its relation to human functioning. He said, "The events of inner experience, as emergent properties of brain processes, became casual constructs with their own laws and dynamics. The whole world of inner experience [must be] recognized and included within the domain of science."

The traditional medical model includes a strong bias toward the "third person" experience of another's presentation. That is to say that although symptoms or the subjective experience of the patient may carry some weight, signs or what can be seen or sensed otherwise in the exterior are thought to be far more valid and reliable.

The "first person" view of disease and dysfunction is often discounted because we have a tendency to have so large an opinion of our own expertise. If this is combined with a low regard for our patient's knowledge, there is little room left for the patient's viewpoint.

We must remember that a patient is not trying to tell us what they think is wrong, but how it feels to be the way that they are. The sensation of living, whether we are healthy or not, can provide valuable information when it is gathered nonjudgmentally and with the respect it deserves.

Thomas Hanna has defined "somatics" as "a field of study dealing with somatic phenomena, i.e., the human being as experienced by himself from the inside." Somatic practitioners not only rely upon their observational skills for diagnoses but also consider the patient's experiences of living as equally significant when planning a regimen of care or assessing progress. Neither the outside nor inside view of the patient is considered necessarily more accurate than the other. Both are subject to misinterpretation and unreliability to the same degree. These problems vary with the complexity of the problem.

The somatic view is essential in the field of physical therapy for reasons obvious to anyone training a patient to move in a new way. The medical world may not appreciate its significance because teaching another to respond to his or her internal sensations may be only as common as the advice to take his or her medication as needed. The goal there is to ablate internal sensation, not expand our awareness of it.

The neurologist Oliver Sacks has written several books on the subject of his patients' inner world. When working to diagnose and treat a variety of disorders he persistently asks the question, "What is it like to be the way you are?" The answers are telling and, at times, remarkably sad. The postencephalatic Parkinsonian says "caged"; the man with a complete loss of short-term memory answers, "I wouldn't say that I feel alive."

When Sacks himself is badly injured he finds it impossible to get his surgeon interested in his sensory agnosia. After all, the surgeon can't see it. He finds help from others who have learned that the inner world of experience has much to do with our functioning. They followed the traditions of therapy that were considered purely intuitive until Sperry proved them both correct and essential to the progression of our art and science in the clinic.

Selected Reading
Hanna T. What is somatics? Part 1. *Somatics*. 1986;5(4).
Sacks O. *A Leg to Stand On*. New York, NY: Summit Books; 1984.

THE PHENOMENAL PERSPECTIVE

I find that if I keep my eyes and ears open I see there are people doing work in this world that is remarkably relevant to the therapy community. Unfortunately, neither we nor they are aware that the other exists and some really fine work may go unnoticed by those who need it the most. In an effort to combat this problem in a small way I want to talk about a newsletter that I've been getting the past couple of years.

Elizabeth A. Behnke is the coordinator of "The Study Project in Phenomenology of the Body." The project works to organize the study of individuals and institutions whose work is relevant to phenomenology of the lived body. Don't worry, I originally didn't have any idea what that might be either.

Phenomenology as a distinct philosophical viewpoint was first described by Edmund Husserl (1895-1938). He basically reflected upon the ways that our communal experiences might be adequately described and developed criteria for the convergence of different sorts of experiences. Behnke describes it more succinctly as "a 20th century approach to the careful study of lived experience as experienced by the experiencer."

I feel this is closely related to the field of "somatics" espoused by Thomas Hanna, the difference being that somatics embraces all living things and phenomenology seems confined to the human experience.

Husserl's remarkably complex thinking is linked to the concrete enterprises of everyday living by the French philosopher Merleau-Ponty (1908-1961). He insisted that our bodies were not objects to be manipulated by some supposed inner ego, but that they are our immediate living presence, not separate from our consciousness but a full accurate expression of what we think. I'm reminded of a con man in the movie "House of Games." He explains to his potential victim that her intentions are always visible somehow, and that this "tell" will always be seen by those of his sort. "The things we want, the things we think, we can do them or not do them, but we can't hide them." The "poker face" of the professional gambler actually extends throughout his body, into the inflection of his voice, and takes years to control. It actually displays a tremendous respect for the teaching of Merleau-Ponty.

A phenomenology of the body would include a wide range of work that examines how it is to be the way we are in the world, and how to describe the experience. To give you some kind of idea of how different subjects of phenomenological perspective can be, consider this: in the Fall 1988 issue under "Works in Progress," Behnke mentions that I am working on a description of the bodily art of juggling (subsequently published in *Jugglers World*) and follows this with Gove's research project on "the psychophysical development of serial killers." Phenomenology has got to be the only thing that these two subjects have in common.

Therapists are often taken to task for inadequate documentation. James Gould wrote "we often write treatment reactions rather than treatment plans." For this we pay with insurance denials and the derision of a physician that can't decipher the purpose of PT. Of course, we have to change our ways if we want to survive in an increasingly socialized system. It's hard though. I think that many clinicians have a natural affinity for the phenomenological viewpoint. This tends to emphasize the subjective experience as described by the patient. As they express themselves with gesture and posture that is as transient as their thoughts and moods, the goniometric measurements so dear to the physician or third-party payer seem inadequate. I'm not suggesting that they aren't necessary.

A favorite theme in phenomenology also relates to the practice of therapy. It is proposed that when we use a tool or other device, getting used to it requires that we "incorporate it into the bulk of our body," that the tool and the person together manifest a "unity of intention."

The people whom we use our tools upon are necessarily shaped by the intended outcome of the tools' properties and ourselves. To come to a patient with either a measuring or therapeutic device changes them and changes us as well. The device and our intention will always limit the patient's response and, possibly, our ability to perceive them. This makes me wary of measurements I must make without my hands and of response to treatment that includes an inanimate machine. I don't think that the issue will ever be resolved. I'm just grateful that so many people are working to explore it.

Selected Reading

Dorko BL. Juggling philosophically. *Jugglers World*. 1989;Spring.

Fisher A. *The Essential Writings of Merleau-Ponty*. New York, NY: Harcourt Brace; 1969.

Gould J. The art of physical therapy. *SOSPT*. 1990;Feb. Editorial.

Lauer TQ. *Phenomenology and the Crises of Philosophy*. New York, NY: Harper & Row; 1965.

THE VISION THING

During the 1988 presidential campaign, George Bush was encouraged by his staff to express his views on the future of our society and its place in global events. "Oh, yeah," he said, "the vision thing." (This is actually true.)

One of the books I found in the pile on my desk is *The Psychology of Perspective and Renaissance Art* by Michael Kubovy. It is a remarkable study of how artists since the early 15th century have dealt with the problems of perspective by the use of various devices and techniques that are evident to only the most knowledgeable observer.

I found it especially interesting to note that correct representation of visual perspective in art is confined to architectural features. The accurate depiction of humans in the same way would result in a grotesque distortion of the cylinders and spheres on which the human form is based. The artist overcomes this by depicting people as if they were simultaneously viewed from two perspectives. This results in our sensation of closeness to the subject while allowing for the clear, naturalistic view that a more distant vantage point would normally afford.

While the device of using multiple perspectives is necessary, it lays bare the problems inherent to any testing we might do that requires "sighting" for symmetry, either of a static body part or the dynamics of its change with movement.

A study by Potter and Rothstein seems to confirm this. In 13 tests of the pelvic region, the 11 that required a visual inspection for symmetry revealed an intertester reliability of less than 50%. The remaining tests required only a subjective report from the patient.

This seems a dramatic example of what can happen when we attempt to use our eyes on the human form as a reliable measure. I wonder at this stage of my career if I should even bother looking at the surface. I know I can't trust my visual perspective.

A detailed study by Patrick A. Heelan takes the problems of visual perception a step further by using a phenomenological view of our visual experience in the world by stating, "...under certain circumstances the shapes of objects that we see fail to match their physical (i.e., third Euclidean) shapes, but instead match certain transforms of those shapes, namely, the appearances the objects would have in a hyperbolic non-Euclidean space." Heelan demonstrates convincingly how such an illusion is depicted by van Gogh's "Bedroom at Arles." At least, it convinced me.

The curved surfaces of the human form appear difficult to see accurately from a single perspective though I have not heard or read much in the therapy literature about the problem. Perhaps it is because, as Kubovy suggests, "...the function of sight is to avoid visual puzzles. When what meets the eye is incomplete or ambiguous, the mind unhesitatingly determines which of the many possible worlds agree most with the data reaching the sense organs."

I look, but have to wonder about the reliability of my tests dependent on what I think I see. I am reminded of asking my wife if the kids need a bath. "Are you crazy?" she asks incredulously, "Just look at them!"

It's funny. They look fine to me. Do you think George and Barbara ever have this problem?

Selected Reading

Heelan PA. *Space Perception and the Philosophy of Science*. Berkeley, Calif: University of California Press; 1983.

Kubovy M. *The Psychology of Perspective and Renaissance Art*. London: Cambridge University Press; 1986.

Potter, Rothstein J. Intertester reliability for selected clinical tests of the sacroiliac joint. *Physical Therapy*. 1985;Nov.

$\mathcal{T}$HE IDEAL BODY

It is rare for any patient to enter treatment without some goals in mind. The therapist as well must have some idea of what the end of care will look like so that they can see that they are headed in the right direction at least.

When we want strength, length, and endurance, these goals are closely associated with each individual's potential. We take into account each patient's age, gender, and size, and the goal for one is often not nearly the same for the next.

But when we feel that the bodily alignment in standing is important for our patient, we usually abandon the concept of individual potential and begin to display our notion of what is ideal. There is a picture on the wall or in a book or in our heads that we want our patients to look like. Usually where they currently are in standing is not straight enough.

This kind of thinking has been identified by Johnson as "Somatic Platonism." He says that the Platonic way of thinking has two qualities:

- The ideal is the same for all
- The ideal is a specifically designed representation, a picture

If Platonism is an idealism of content or image that ignores process or function, it will strictly limit any therapist that depends upon it. I was never in the service, but I have been told that the prolonged position of attention, while looking good, was not accompanied by comfort or easy breathing, especially while being berated by a superior.

The plumb line used to determine how far we may deviate from ideal posture measures our functioning in no significant way. It only exposes us as remarkably pliable beings that may function with exquisite precision and grace despite our persistent movement from some transient though ideal position.

Among Johnson's objections to Platonism as applied to body position are that the ideal model will always devalue the patient's current reality and that the therapist's perceptions and approach to care will become limited.

The first of these objections strikes me as psychologically significant in any clinical setting. If the patients are simply shown how they deviate from what they should be, they may become inappropriately dependent upon the therapist for guidance. I'd much prefer that patients use me as a resource who helps them understand the solution to their problems lie within themselves. It will emerge, and improvement will be a natural consequence of the work. Remember, I'm talking about posture here.

Using an ideal model for posture would surely limit my perception of my patients if I hold not only the perfect image in my head but also the image of typical dysfunction. If I adhere to an image of ideal position, I must of necessity create models of common aberration. In the interest of time I will probably begin to assume that movement from the ideal has taken place in a typical fashion. This bias is a natural consequence of Platonism in posture and I've fallen into its trap more than once.

Perhaps the most insidious effect of Somatic Platonism is the way that our care proceeds when the goal includes the chosen ideal. Ideals are simply not attainable. The posture humans choose is remarkably transient and the path from one to another is as individual as our personal gestures. When we discard the notion that postural training ends up looking like some particular image, we can begin to provide each patient with companionship along their unique path toward improved functioning.

<u>Selected Reading</u>
Johnson D. Somatic platonism. *Somatics*. 1980;3(1).

CHARCOT'S LAMENT

In 1872, Charcot wondered how Duchenne had suddenly "discovered" muscular dystrophy when it had probably been displayed to every physician beginning with Hippocrates. He wrote, "Why do we have to go over the same set of symptoms 20 times before we understand it? Why does the first statement of what seems a new fact always leave us cold? [It is] because our minds have to take in something that deranges our original set of ideas, but we are all of us like that in this miserable world."

This is clearly a lament to which many clinicians can relate. The excitement of sudden realization that what is now a perfectly obvious sign of specific dysfunction is usually tempered with an internal sense that you should have understood this sooner.

I'm pretty sure that much of what I see quite clearly in my patients today was there when I was a student 20 years ago. My eyesight was actually better then (I had more hair, too), but I couldn't see what was in front of me. Like all of us, my perceptual clarity improved over time with repetition and knowledge.

How does this happen?

The neurologist Oliver Sacks recently published *Seeing Voices, A Journey Into the World of the Deaf*. He writes extensively of the mental transition that a congenitally deaf person must make while learning sign language in infancy. After many repetitions they realize that gestures can represent other things. This is thought to be a part of our genetically acquired general linguistic competence, something the hearing do naturally with the sound of words. However, the grammatical structure of sign (or spoken language for that matter) is an example of "epigenesis," a form of learning that actually evolves within us as we grow. Edelman calls this process neuronal group selection or "neural Darwinism." It is characterized by a selection of neuronal networks that form in direct response to environmental pressure. What we eventually recognize and understand depends upon what we've experienced repetitively and within a certain context.

The acquisition of sign among the congenitally deaf is a dramatic example of neural Darwinism in action. It is especially distinctive because it is in a visual mode. Something repetitively seen suddenly acquires a new meaning.

The relation of this work to assessment in therapy is evident when you consider the fact that the ability to finally recognize elements in our environment is usually dependent upon the repetition of a sensory/motor act on our part each time a stimulus is within our awareness. A therapist not only sees something but usually has a tactile sense of it as well. Many accurate diagnoses are made without ever actually hearing of a symptom that would specifically identify the dysfunction. Like the deaf, we must interpret what we see and feel without the benefit of any sound (i.e., a specific complaint) to lead us to our conclusion. Our ability to connect the patient's physical presentation to an underlying process that we cannot see or hear evolves over time with repeated exposure and the acquisition of our own tactile skills. Charcot's lament is a bit off the mark. His frustration at not being able to immediately recognize every new thing before him is just a pessimistic way of viewing the way we learn.

When clinicians finally begin to see their patients clearly, they realize that often the most important aspects of disability are hidden because of their simplicity and familiarity. The price of accurate assessment is always vigilance. If you ever stop watching carefully, nothing new will appear.

Selected Reading

Edelman G. *Neural Darwinism*. New York, NY: Basic Books; 1987.
Rosenfeld J. *The Invention of Memory*. New York, NY: Basic Books; 1988.
Sacks O. *Seeing Voices, A Journey Into the World of the Deaf*. Berkeley, Calif:
    University of California Press; 1989.

My FATHER'S NECK

A sudden onset of transient but sharp cervical pain began in my father last year. This was followed by bouts of dizziness that had both his physician and I concerned.

I had not helped him with his discomfort despite my best efforts to magically fix him after the occasional Sunday dinner. This usually works with other relatives.

His doctor cleaned his ears and sent him for a MRI. Dad said the test was like having a jackhammer next to his head. It was negative.

He went for more testing through an ENT man. He watched lights fly across his visual field and listened to a wide variety of sounds. Finally, he lay supine and let his neck extend completely over the end of a table. The technician blew blasts of cold air in his ears and questioned him about his reactions.

The varieties of testing that are available in medicine today display the progression of scientific thought. Remember that science is not a collection of facts but rather a way of looking at things. Many tests help us see some part of the system that is hidden from our sensory apparatus. Ideally, testing reveals the patient to him- or herself.

Testing does not just ask questions. It usually provides stimulation of some sort. The sound of the MRI disturbed my father and made him want to escape. The auditory testing he found interesting. He sang professionally "by ear" for many years and as the testing revealed his acute sense of pitch, it drew him in. His verbal description of the two tests is accompanied by an unconscious posturing that reveals his experience beyond words.

Our body parts do not react universally to stimuli in some strictly proportional relation. This is to say that we are nonlinear beings and what is irritating to some is positively therapeutic to others. It also means that strong stimulation at times produces a small response and a gentle nudge may waken a variety of processes both sequentially and concurrently.

I have stood for an hour in line with hundreds of others at an amusement park waiting to be tossed about, turned upside down, and spun around and paid for the privilege. Is such an experience therapeutic? Why else would people flock to it? If the ride suddenly shuts down, there is great disappointment and a sense of loss in the gathered crowd.

I have got to believe that at least some of the people in this line have the kind of chronically recurrent spinal pain that sends them to my office for gentle movement and carefully chosen resting postures. A small slip in the kitchen would set their recovery back 6 weeks.

If the stimulation of the roller coaster is therapeutic, I think it is more so for those people who choose to accept it as it comes, without resistance. They are the ones with their hands up in the air.

All the tests my father went through were negative. I never really treated him nor did anyone else. He gave himself up to the testing and has felt fine ever since.

Next Sunday I am supposed to take a look at my Aunt Ann.

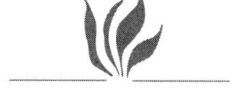

THE GRAND CANYON

I took my family to the Grand Canyon this past summer. When you first drive up to the south rim, there is a place you can park and walk to peer over the edge.

My first thought there remains today: "There's no point in taking a photo, the best part of this can't be seen, only felt. And the feeling can only occur as I stand here at the rim."

S. Kay Toombs, writer and multiple sclerosis patient, states in the introduction of her book, "[My] inability to communicate with my doctor does not result from inattentiveness or insensitivity but from fundamental disagreement about the nature of illness. Rather than representing a shared reality between us, illness represents two quite distinct realities: the meaning of one being significantly and distinctly different from the meaning of another."

Using a remarkably intricate but precise argument, Toombs traces the problems with patient/doctor dialogue to the fact that they are talking about two entirely different things: the lived experience of a life disrupted by illness on the one hand, and an objective disease state on the other.

I often wonder where I stand as a therapist in the midst of this, but I guess it probably varies.

Perhaps if I return to my thoughts about how it felt to stand at the rim of that canyon, I can get a better feel for this relationship.

If I imagine the patient as the one on the rim, struck as I was by a distinct disruption of my usual vision and experience, while the physician and I live some distance from there, this dialogue comes to me:

Patient: "Hey, come here and look at this, it's like nothing I've ever seen before."

Physician: "I really don't have the time right now. Anyway, I've seen plenty of photos of this view so I know what you're talking about."

Patient: "No, no, you don't understand. It's not just what you can see, it's a sensation I can't describe. You have to be with me to know what I mean."

Therapist: "I've got a little time, maybe we can look at this together."

I know that it's perfectly possible to practice therapy in a way that never brings you to a place that allows you to sense the patient's experience. It's even easier to practice medicine that way. Every time I step to the rim with a patient, I have to keep in mind that his or her physician has probably not done the same.

When I speak to physicians about what I've seen in patients and why I treated them in unexpected ways, it is no wonder they don't understand me. Every day can contain indescribable moments like that view of the canyon.

You have to be there.

Selected Reading

Toombs SK. *The Meaning of Illness: A Phenomenological Account of the Different Perspectives of Physician and Patient.* Dordiecht: Kluwer; 1992.

WHY DON'T THEY HURT?

*"I haven't got time for the pain, I haven't the need for the pain,
I haven't the use for the pain."*

Carly Simon

My father has been bowlegged all my life. He was 35 when I was born and I'm sure the genu varum so easily seen in him today was evident long before then.

X-rays taken 3 years ago reveal no cartilage and severe degenerative changes. If you showed these to many physicians they would guess that his function was markedly decreased by pain and restricted mobility.

But Dad walks about in comfort most of the time. A couple of injections in the past 10 years resolved some transient inflammation and at 79 he stills carries his large frame step over step several times each day, up and down, to and from his basement office.

I realize that asking the question; "Why don't his knees hurt more than they do?" is not really fair. It is much like asking someone to prove that there is no Santa Claus.

But this issue of no pain despite plenty of perfectly good reasons to hurt haunts me. If the care I provide for others begins in my understanding of what pathology brings, and what I can do to combat that, I can't help but wonder why in this instance the expected complaint is absent.

In *The Culture of Pain*, David Morris contends that pain is not properly considered a sensation, but a perception. Thus its presence is connected to the rest of our lives.

My tendency when faced with something mysterious is to consider its multiple implications and think of what not knowing everything might have to teach me about myself. The mystery of my father's flexible, painless knees leads me to this:

Dad descends to the basement each day to attend to a part of his life most people never express. Here he writes poetry that celebrates the accomplishments of others or his feelings about a variety of things. These poems are eventually published in local papers, read aloud at ceremonies, and printed on cards to be dispersed throughout the community.

You might say that Dad depends upon his legs to get him where he needs to go in order to do something unique, creative, and close to his heart. For all I know, without making this trip with regularity the past 40 years his heart might have broken, and his knees might have felt and behaved as expected.

In a poem about personal desire and creative energy, David Whyte says:

Always this energy smolders inside
when it remains unlit
the body fills with dense smoke

Maybe people with reason to hurt don't hurt because somehow in their life what would be painful otherwise is channeled into something else unique to them, something creative and full of their inner life. Maybe that's why my father's knees carry him to this task each day, refusing to demand rest and not bothering him with their pain.

<u>Selected Reading</u>
Morris D. *The Culture of Pain.* Berkeley, Calif: University of California Press; 1991.
Whyte D. Out on the ocean. *Songs for Coming Home.* Many Rivers Press; 1989.

THE LADY IN THE LACE GLOVES

I had a new patient come to my office on a weekday morning. Her complaint of pain was recent and as yet it hadn't significantly interfered with her work.

A professional woman in her mid-40s, she held a very responsible position and administrated the work of a large staff while having established a private consulting business on the side.

Her outward appearance struck me as remarkably incongruent to the time of day. She wore a perfectly tailored black skirt and matching top. Over this was a jacket with wide sleeves and collar, both trimmed generously with feathery, black fake fur that floated like an aura extending from her surface as she walked toward me. She was in the process of removing a beautiful pair of lace gloves. It was a cold November day.

There are many things we learn on the job that can't possibly be included in our schooling or apprenticeship. I knew when I shook this woman's hand that I wasn't going to help her. It was the kind of knowledge won over 20 years in the clinic, and I pay close attention to it.

I don't currently have a problem with chronic pain, nor have I ever. I am mindful of Lorenzo Milan's admonition that I am among the "temporarily able-bodied," however, and I try to prepare for what may come my way. I have also freely chosen to work in a profession expected to understand and assist those with pain. I feel their pain and the consequences of disability from the "outside-in" as yet; someday that may change.

Having said that, I want to talk about what I know that led me to despair of ever helping this patient.

I know that physical pain treatable with conservative care in my office requires some measure of "somatic authenticity." You're not going to read this phrase anywhere else, because I just made it up.

Somatic authenticity is the bodily expression of our desire to move unencumbered by cultural expectations, external direction, or willful intent. It requires us to relinquish posing and posturing and accept unconscious motivation as that which is needed for improvement.

In the movie "The Remains of the Day," Anthony Hopkins portrays an English butler extraordinaire. His manner, speech, and dress are impeccable, and he has accepted his feudal position to such a degree that he will not even attend to his dying father a few rooms away because it would disrupt his duties at an important dinner party.

This character has come to believe that what he presents to the world (his persona) is all that he is. There is no room in his life for any kind of expression other than service or house management. He pays dearly for this with a life devoid of passion or spontaneity.

The butler and my patient had a lot in common. I spent an hour with her and she made some effort to be nice in return, but only in a Cruella DeVille kind of way.

I didn't help her and a few days later she called to ask for her referral so that she might see another therapist.

I feel a little uneasy about judging this patient so quickly, but we parted on friendly terms. As I watched her float out the door, I couldn't help but wonder how long a journey this patient had just begun.

Selected Reading
Milam L. *Crip Zen: A Manual for Survivors*. Mho and Mho Works; 1993.

+OW DID I GET LIKE THIS?

Once a therapist explains to a patient what is thought to be wrong, he or she knows what is coming next.

"How did I get like this?"

It is a tough question. The complex and chaotic nature of life makes it impossible to account for all the things that might produce what we finally see in our office.

At a conference on posture in Canada, I heard a fellow speaker describe "intrauterine packing syndrome." This occurs when a large first-born baby or one of a multiple birth is compressed during pregnancy for lack of space.

I listened absently for awhile. It was late in the day and this sounded like just some more useless information that had nothing to do with clinical reality. Then something started to wake up in the deeper recesses of my mind.

The ultimate expression of these compressive forces is a postural deviation I have seen many times—right hip external rotation and abduction with relative internal rotation on the left, left tibial internal rotation, right calcaneal valgus, left forefoot adductus.

This is me. I have invested a lot of time and effort observing this pattern in my own body and I am convinced that I have done all that I can do with the tissues available for me to change. Stretching the connective tissue and regular coordinative exercise of the leg and foot have certainly enhanced my tolerance for activity but the bony orientation never corrects beyond a certain point. It doesn't feel like it is going to get any better.

According to Breig and Troup, internal rotation of the hip will reduce the adaptive potential of the nervous tissue ipsilaterally. My left side certainly has a tendency for trouble. It talks to me, and I have learned to respect its limits.

How did I get like this? Is it possible that my current state has its origins much further back than my last heavy lift or the way I slept last night? Can I answer these questions for a relative stranger when I do not know myself that well?

Fortunately, my maturation as a therapist includes an increasing tolerance for ambiguity and acceptance of the fact that we cannot always know the answers to some perfectly reasonable questions.

I am a twin, and although my sister Leah in Philadelphia certainly does not crowd me as she once probably did (or I her), we remain connected in the unique way twins do. It may be difficult to describe in words, but I think sometimes that I still feel it.

Selected Reading
Breig A, Troup J. Biomechanical considerations in the straight-leg-raising test. *Spine.* 1979;4(3).

Suggested Reading
Dorko B. A simple test of autonomic balance. *PT Forum.* 1989;8(28).

POSING

I just returned from a sitting with the photographer and I'm anxious to see how I look.

Of course, I suppose I could just look in a mirror. After all, I'm wearing the same tie and my hair is still combed.

But I know that I am not quite the same just now as I will appear in the photo. I was perched on a stool holding my coat flat against me to eliminate wrinkles. I held my chin down, my head tilted just so, and was told to think of something pleasant as I smiled. (Don't ask).

I guess I looked pretty good. I know that I felt awful. Within 30 seconds of sitting down on the stool my left lower thorax began to ache. It wasn't anything severe. I knew it would pass once I shifted position, but that was now up to the photographer. Our mutual concern with my appearance overrode my desire to grimace, to express my discomfort without actually whining.

How many times do therapists ask the patient to pose? When we place them against a grid on the wall and encourage them to get their various parts lined up, is it possible similar discomfort might show up eventually? If we assume that there is a direct correlation between muscular strength and joint position, then we are not reading the literature. If I assume that muscular weakness is in some way painful, then I've just created a relationship between function and pain that is not substantiated in the literature I've read.

So why do I hurt? Simply put, I have deformed my system beyond its adaptive potential. I rarely feel this in my life despite a good deal of vigorous exercise. The element added to my movement today was that of posing.

I looked up pose in the dictionary: "to strike an attitude for effect, to pretend to be what one is not."

I recently treated a competitive diver. This young lady began competing years ago in gymnastics. She lies supine as if prepared to begin a routine or run to the end of the diving board. Such a posture requires work enough in standing and even more when lying down. She expresses no awareness that she holds herself so carefully and getting her to change toward authentic rest has been very difficult. After all, her appearance has been rated numerically by judges for years. No wonder she hurts.

If you add an "i" to pose you get poise: "balance and stability, ease and dignity of manner, self-assurance, composure." It would be nice to appear poised. If I can get my patients to achieve this, I will be doing some wonderful therapy.

Maybe my next photo session will be less painful if I just remember to add that "i" to the sitting.

Selected Reading
Rothstein J. *APTA Journal.* 1990;Aug. Editorial.

THE PIANO LESSON

In the mid-morning my mother sits in her chair, hot tea at hand, her collection of books about Harry Truman on the shelf behind her. Earlier in the kitchen, before breakfast, she had asked where she should sit.

"Right here, as usual," I said. She looked at me, "Nothing is usual around here."

Indeed, she is more often confused than not and speaks little except to agree with my father or comment tersely in a variety of ways that she doesn't remember recent events and is not sure about the present. As I watch her sitting silently, she appears to be listening to something and the fingers of her right hand move in a precise and intricate pattern across her knee.

At the 1993 APTA convention in Cincinnati, I noticed an increasing gap in our profession. It is not simply a split between the research and clinical communities. These are not mutually exclusive. It is a split between therapists who refuse to ignore subtle, but persistent, clinical phenomena, perhaps impossible to measure, and those who insist nothing can be said to exist without exhaustive study. The latter group tends to make fun of the former.

At the Catherine Worthingham Fellow Forum I heard Helen Hislop, PhD, PT, define science as "moral imagination." That phrase was just one of many she used, but it was the one I felt I should write down.

The highly respected psychoanalyst James Hillman states, "The primary function of the human being is to imagine. [Psychology works] not by suppressing our madness, but rather by forming it. And form means art. Art as formed madness."

Hillman says nothing about imagination having a "moral" quality. Is "immoral" imagination unscientific?

As a physical, rather than a psycho, therapist, I am accustomed to watching bodily expression. I am trained to note postural habits, dysfunctional movement, weakness, and facilitation.

It is when I start to note unconsciously motivated movement seemingly unrelated to disability and wonder aloud what it may signify that I invite the derision of some of my colleagues. The unique, artful expressions of the body that make us human cannot be measured or easily interpreted. No graph can contain them, no normative values can be assigned to them. And my failing as a serious researcher probably lies in the fact that I cannot ignore them.

I asked my mother if she was playing the piano. She smiled, laughed a little, and said yes, stopping for a few moments before returning to complete the piece, some tune learned decades ago and uniquely expressed through her hands. Hands that never forget.

The therapist in me wonders what this movement provides her that no amount of exercise, positioning, or manual care could. Perhaps she is in some fashion growing younger through her body though her faculties age.

I doubt that such speculation is scientifically defensible in the strictest sense, but I can't help but wonder what my mother is trying to teach me.

Selected Reading

Hillman J, Ventura M. *We've Had One Hundred Years of Psychotherapy and the World Is Getting Worse.* San Francisco, Calif: Harper; 1992.

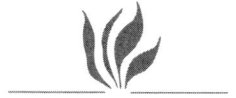

WHERE ARE YOU?

You keep thinking of pain as a place you could leave, walk out and slam the last heavy door. But the pain you inhabit is a region, only your own, a place where your memories happen, a room no one else can come into, however close they try to stand.

Adapted from "Pointing to the Place of the Pain" by Karen Fiser

I'm well aware of the fact that the phrase "functional capacity" is a sacred icon in the world of rehabilitation in general and physical therapy in particular. I know that objective measures form the bulk of data in outcomes research. I read constantly of how if we don't prove what we do actually alters patients, something dreadful will happen to our income. I know, I know, I know.

But each day I see patients with absolutely no interest in their functioning beyond normal sleep, prolonged sitting, or a walk through the mall. They just want to escape the pain or have me take it away or learn some magic movement that will relieve it. Each day those of us working alone without the support of rehab services must address the immediate concerns of the patient. They haven't read the books on functional assessment or the studies proving that pain levels and activity levels are unrelated. For the most part, they don't come in wanting to look better, they want to feel it.

A major issue to every patient is the location of their pain. They assume that this is very important to me, and who could blame them? Their doctor wants to know and all the other therapists asked. They've always had this spot prodded before and modalities of every sort have been concentrated there.

But as Gregory Grieve points out, referred pain occurs in the body image somewhere in the CNS. It never follows the distribution of a major nerve trunk. It never corresponds to the overlying dermatome. And it never follows the pattern of the vascular tree. Given this, you have to wonder why we pay so much attention to its location. Maybe we're asking the wrong questions.

Let me shift gears here.

Each Tuesday evening I walk down a street in Kent, Ohio on my way to a harmonica lesson. Two doors from the music store is a tattoo parlor. It's always busy and in warm weather the open door emits a high-pitched buzzing that goes through my head like a nail.

I have no desire to stop and get a tattoo. I can't even conjure up an image of what design might be permanently acceptable to me. But beyond that, I would have a terrible time deciding where on my body I would like to put it. I would literally have to decide where to hurt. It's a choice I have never made before.

I know the pain of tattooing is not great and doesn't last. But I look at the people waiting inside that door and think of how different they are from my patients. They're willing to trade a little discomfort for a chance to express something. Something that will always be there. Similarly, my harmonica in my pocket, I'm headed toward another sort of unique expression that requires effort and endless repetition.

We don't originally get to choose where to hurt. We can at best only choose how to view our pain, how to see its relation to our lives.

Chronic pain chooses us. And its presence cannot be adequately pointed at or shaded in on a chart. It is a region we come to occupy and perceive differently each day.

Maybe the therapist should not always ask, "Where do you hurt?" but occasionally, "Where are you today?"

Selected Reading

Fiser K. Pointing to the place of the pain. *Words Like Fate and Pain.* Cambridge, Mass: Zoland Books; 1992.

Grieve GP. Scrutinizing tacit assumptions in manual therapy. *Journal of Manual and Manipulative Therapy.* 1993;1(4).

BACKACHES AND EARTHQUAKES

I understand that in Japan there are 200 seismographic reporting stations continuously monitoring and analyzing the earth's activity. In January 1995 they told the people of Kobe: "Hey, you guys just had a major earthquake." And the people of Kobe responded from beneath the rubble: "No kidding?"

Often a patient will recount the visit to the doctor that preceded coming to see me: "He examined me very thoroughly, poked all around my spine, checked my reflexes, and asked a lot of questions. Then he told me I had a backache."

I know that preventive care is a popular and logical way to use our current medical knowledge. Studies have long shown that certain behaviors help us withstand future stresses on our body or retard the growth of unhealthy processes. But the distinction between prevention and prediction becomes obvious in a situation like the one in Japan.

All of the effort put into building things that could theoretically withstand the stresses of internal disruption and all the monitoring of activity beneath the surface did not help to predict when some significant change would occur. This is as true of our bodies as it is of the earth beneath us.

Nor does prevention necessarily mean we will easily withstand future injury. Illnesses can expose our inherent weaknesses like the earthquake destroyed entirely the wooden houses of Kobe. Each of us has vulnerable parts that are unique to our lives and impossible to strengthen or constantly protect. Achilles remained vulnerable at his heel because that is where his mother continued to hold him (read the story) and there was no escaping that.

Can we predict a future backache? Well, a recent study by Newton and Waddell suggests that even the most sophisticated isokinetic testing has proven unreliable when used in pre-employment screening. Of course, certain manufacturers will take issue with this, but they must be reminded of their vested interest in any evaluation of their product. Newton's analysis of 108 articles, many published by proponents of isokinetic trunk testing, reveals what most researchers know: What we see and report depends partly on what is there and partly on who is looking.

I wonder what would happen if the people who sold earthquake insurance were also in charge of interpreting seismographs? Something tells me the tendency to predict trouble would become more frequent. The postural screening booth I see a local chiropractor set up in the mall might have a similar effect.

Maybe our attempts at predicting backache are connected to our very human desire to know something about the future. With science, we have accomplished this with eclipses of the sun and the gender of our unborn children. But when it comes to the future of human behavior and our subsequent health, we haven't been as successful. It looks like the earth's future behavior is as much a mystery, and the absolute absence of warning in Japan proved that again.

Selected Reading
Newton M, Waddell G. Trunk strength testing with iso-machines. *Spine*. 1993;18(7).

HIS FATHER'S VOICE

My Father

My office is in the cellar of my home,
and I am working late.
Mother and father are coming to visit for the night.
I hear my father's voice above.
Oh, how I love that voice.
For all that is broken with fathers and sons
and with this father and this son,
that voice,
it comforts me
and cradles my core.

Michael Dwinell

There is a recording of his father's voice in a desk drawer at home, and Tom Bear has no way of hearing it.

I have lunch with Tom a couple times each week, and despite the fact that he is an orthopedist, we get along remarkably well. Our topics of conversation have an amazing range and are punctuated with laughter. Over the years we've watched each other mature as men and clinicians and now we listen to each other speak of the demise of health care as we had hoped to practice it. We have no illusions about fixing this, but it helps to talk.

I mentioned a new book to him: Clifford Stoll's *Silicon Snake Oil: Second Thoughts on the Information Highway.* In one chapter Stoll points out that storing anything for future retrieval requires the invention of a format, literally a shape that can then somehow be read and translated to a form we can understand. The latest format we are generally familiar with is the compact disc and the advantages it offers have revolutionized the computer and music industries.

Stoll points out that although CDs may have decades if not centuries of life in them, this is not what determines their future usefulness, it's the reading mechanism.

My brother Kevin owns a collection of 78 rpm albums. They are carefully stored and perfectly sound but there is one little problem: he has no place to play them. That is to say he no longer owns a turntable that will turn at this rate and those that exist are increasingly rare and expensive.

I told Tom at lunch it had occurred to me that each of us individually is a format containing our history in the form of shape and size and tendencies to behave. The reading mechanisms designed to measure and decipher all of that information have become increasingly sophisticated (x-rays, EMGs, CT scans, MRIs, etc.) although our format remains the same. Unlike the audio or computer industries where changes in reading mechanisms have made some formats obsolete, the health industry strives to create new reading mechanisms for the same format. Clearly this is a testament to human complexity.

Tom said he can see that the insurance industry is beginning to eliminate the reading mechanism we call the doctor by no longer asking for a second opinion but only an MRI after a single physical exam. This despite the false negatives and positives known to occur with such tests. "They don't want my opinion, they want the machine's," he says.

Francis Bear's voice was imprinted on a "wire" recording back in the late 1940s. These preceded the magnetic tape most of us know. He died when Tom was 11 years old, and hearing that voice again would be a wonderful thing if only there were some way.

But I've heard Francis's voice. Tom spoke to me one day of how his father had taught him to pour oil from a can without spilling a drop, and of how he passed this specific skill on to his son. Listening to him speak and pantomime the movement, I learned myself. Perhaps we should remember that as humans we are formats, reading mechanisms, and pretty good recorders as well. When Tom tells me of something that his father once said, those words contain a human quality that only his son can give them, and although the wire recording might be more objective in a sense, I don't feel it would be more authentic.

The move away from human reading mechanisms requested by the insurance companies is predictable, cost-conscious, and sad all at once. What we end up with is often like that recording in the drawer. It is not the essence of the man, and it gives us little insight into what he was about. That recording is in Tom. And sometimes he plays it for me at lunch.

Selected Reading
Dwinell M. My father. *The Best of Pilgrimage*. Vol 1. 1986-1992.
Stoll C. *Silicon Snake Oil: Second Thoughts on the Information Highway*. New York, NY: Doubleday; 1995.

TELLING THE TALE

"All the higher processes of art are the processes of simplification."

Willa Cather

*L*et me begin this by saying that when the musician Danny Gatton, died it was reported in both Time *and* Newsweek. *In other words, Danny Gatton was Somebody, even though I had never heard of him. I discovered him during his obituary on National Public Radio reported by one of its regular correspondents who was also Gatton's personal friend.*

The reporter spoke of Gatton's astounding virtuosity on the guitar, the speed and intricacy of the riffs he could play in any style, and of his failure to become a commercial success despite his many years of effort and the unqualified admiration of his peers.

A popular performer in clubs around Washington DC, Gatton remarked near the end of his life that he wanted to "play less." But by this he didn't mean fewer performances, he meant fewer notes. One of his last recordings included Brian Wilson's "In My Room" played slowly and simply. It was Gatton's favorite cut from that album.

I have the impression that I am commonly successful with my patients these days, although I would be hard-pressed to prove that to the satisfaction of certain researchers. What I mean is that people of many sorts enter the clinical milieu of my office with only the story of their pain, and they eventually leave with a story of their recovery as well. If they don't know that second story, I haven't succeeded, and that's relatively rare.

If I can recall accurately the nature of my early days in practice when what I did or said seemed ineffective or inconsequential in many cases,

I can see now that the major element missing compared to today was the use of story. I've always had some knowledge and skill, but early on I had no effective way of imparting these to others or hearing their response in ways that were meaningful. I made speeches, and I expected speeches in return.

Somehow, probably as the end result of failure and the wandering toward other methods of care it produces, I began to use metaphor whenever possible. And I started to hear the stories of others.

An effective story deepens our understanding of what we feel is happening and allows us to attach some meaning to otherwise trivial or even painful events. When it includes images that make us realize we are not alone in our personal dilemma, and certainly not the first to face it, the story becomes therapy.

The relation of story to poetry lies in its metaphorical, experiential, and simplistic stylings. The metaphors help us see in familiar images otherwise invisible processes and situations. Briggs points out that "poetry isn't explaining experience, it is a state of experiencing." And in the simple lines, plots, and characters a story describes, the chaos and complexity of our life itself is reduced to something manageable.

When I heard the story of Danny Gatton's life and death (of a self-inflicted gunshot wound) at 49, I saw that my own maturation as a therapist has always included a reduction in speech and an enhancement of story. Gatton wanted to play fewer notes, but his technical skills seemed to have overwhelmed him, and his public was not interested in the simple style he desired. I want to speak less, and I want to more accurately interpret the small gestures, comments, and descriptions people bring with them and cannot hide.

The following essays display the use of story, stories people have brought to me and stories I bring to them. Without question they are among the most popular among my readers, and I feel my growth as a clinician was greatest when I discovered them.

Selected Reading

Briggs J, Monaco R. *Metaphor: The Logic of Poetry.* New York, NY: Pace University Press; 1990.

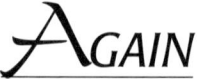GAIN

"I do not believe that sheer suffering teaches. If suffering alone taught, then all the world would be wise, since everyone suffers. To suffering must be added mourning, understanding, patience, love, openness, and the willingness to remain vulnerable."

Anne Morrow Lindbergh

In this business of physical therapy, we are often only vaguely aware of the nature and treatment of conditions that some of our colleagues deal with each day. Specialization does this, and it's unavoidable.

In my generation we were not personally familiar with the treatment of polio and its victims, but almost all of my teachers had lived and worked through the epidemic 40 years ago. I've come to understand that this work formed them in ways that were both hard and soft, and I feel that some of the "warrior" mentality that pervades today's care is a remnant of successful strategies for polio, even if we are clearly treating entirely different problems. Right or wrong, the legacy of therapy's role in polio still affects us and it won't soon leave.

In fact, it is returning.

People who had recovered from paralysis years ago are now experiencing a return of the weakness, exhaustion, and pain that surrounded them as children. And this time, fighting physically against it seems not to help.

The most popular theory explaining post-polio syndrome proposes that the motor neurons that had been trained and forced to support the muscle cells that their stricken neighbors could no longer feed are now wearing out. They've been asked to do too much and now they demand rest. When evaluation reveals weakness, rest is prescribed, not exactly something physical therapists are used to doing.

It is said that when a myth or story is entirely understood, when it loses its mystery, it will die. It will not be passed on to the next generation unless some aspect maintains multiple meanings or details that invite speculation, imagination, and unique interpretation.

When a song, a painting, or a poem remains present and seemingly new year after year, it is because it has something more to teach us, yet always remains mysterious in some way.

It could be argued that polio built our profession. If this were true, its demise might somehow diminish our standing, but that's a stretch, and just a bit too romantic a view of therapy for me.

The truth is this: Polio has resurfaced in its original form in some isolated areas and its old victims are now being reminded of its presence once again.

I was struck by a quote from a woman again weakened into immobility after years of independence: "Many of us never got the chance to mourn our losses. It's important for people with post-polio to face their experience, allow themselves to feel sad."

The biologic theories of recurrence make sense to me and I suppose that they are correct. But I have to wonder why this wasn't foreseen, and what we might learn now that the disease is returning to a new generation of therapists.

This story is very much alive.

Selected Reading
Elmer-Dewit P. Reliving polio. *Time*. 1994;Mar 28.

THE STORY

"My grandfather was beating my grandmother so severely that the doctor intervened. He told her to leave him before he killed her. And she did."

Sitting at the breakfast table in my mother's kitchen I listened to this story again as I have several times the past few months. My mother will turn 80 years old soon and is not aware of the day of the week or who she has spoken to recently. But she remembers this story and has been recounting it in this spare, terse way with increasing frequency.

I wonder, "Why this story these days?" She has many others to tell, stories with humor and warmth.

In a recent article by Naomi Feil it is suggested that a story will be repeated until its meaning is clear. Only by looking at the details and implications of the event recounted might we discover why the unconscious has chosen this story to emerge again and again. Feil suggests we "validate" the storyteller with attention and empathy so that some resonance and communication might occur.

Sam Keen and Anne Valley-Fox write in *Your Mythic Journey*, "To be a person is to have a story to tell...find the unconscious and make it conscious. [But,] you can't tell who you are unless someone is listening."

I began to wonder about the implications of my great-grandmother's decision to leave. This must have been about 1890 and she had seven children. The youngest son was my grandfather, Will Hinske.

These days my mother is losing conscious contact with her immediate past and increasingly her childhood memories as well. She remembers her father though, and he was undoubtedly the central figure in her life. She remembers too her years of working as a nurse. When she graduated from high school her mother forbade her the nurse's training she desired and she had to wait until she had raised six children and was 48 years old before beginning her education. It was her life's work and nothing, I mean nothing, was going to stop her.

The psychologist James Hillman speaks of desire as that which we cannot buy. It's not in the mall, and we don't simply ask for what we desire, we move toward it. My mother's desire to be a caregiver is a good example of "personal mythology," the examination of our lives in order to discover how they are unique and what they mean. Fulfilling work is that which is part of our personal myth. There is no history of medical training in my mother's family. Her father drove a laundry truck, owned and rented property, and prospered. His older brother, visibly damaged by their father, helped out. My mother has never recounted the story of her grandmother without mentioning the doctor, the caregiver, that saved them with some simple but difficult advice. She acknowledges that her desire to nurse came from this man, and no longer repeats the story.

I used to wonder what brought me to therapy and always felt empty when it was suggested that I liked to help others. I know that I followed my mother to the hospital for reasons more profound, reasons that began with an event in the last century, and are found in a story only my mother's aging has allowed her to tell.

Selected Reading

Feil N. Validation therapy. *Somatics*. 1991-1992;8(3).
Keen S, Valley-Fox A. *Your Mythic Journey*. Los Angeles, Calif: Tarcher; 1989.

PAIN AND MEANING

"Dad can't get out of bed, his back hurts him."

My brother is calling me at my office at 7:15 a.m. Two hours later I walk into my father's bedroom where he lies supine, perfectly still, his large hands across his barrel chest. "Hi Barry." He sounds fragile and exhausted.

His right calf had been swelling recently and some sharp pain had been transient there. I had helped him with a shoulder and neck pain the previous week, and this had not returned. But this morning he felt a vise-like spasm in his low back and simply could not move.

As I employed manual care as best I could, he began to speak of the last time he felt a pain like this.

"I was 19 and was the helper on a beer truck. We had to carry the kegs into the bars, up and down stairs to the cellar. And my driver, well...it was my job. I woke up one morning and couldn't move, just like this. I called for my mother, but she was down in the kitchen and couldn't hear me. Finally, I rolled out of the bed and landed on the floor. My mother heard that and she ran upstairs, saw me, and said in Slovak, 'don't move.' She tore the bed sheets in long strips and bound my torso around and around, tying and pinning it at my side. And then she just..."

My father raised his arms as if lifting something and when his hands rose to his head he began to sob. A deep cry of frustration and sorrow.

My mother remained near and clearly understood that my father was not well, but was unable to do more than adjust his blanket or hold his hand. She couldn't explain the situation to my sister on the phone. Although her feelings are clear, words don't come easily to her any-more.

My dad had just spent a month planning a family reunion. His six children are scattered. My family is no different from others in our need to see each other and, in truth, we do not come together without pal-pable friction and the real possibility of old wounds being opened. It had not been a time without some difficult moments.

Dad now cares daily for his widowed older sister and admits it is wearing at times. He is 76 and says to me this morning, "What is hap-pening to this body?"

We got him to the hospital where some evidence of a blood clot in his leg made admission necessary. His back pain was very much a secondary concern and although transferring him to the x-ray table was very painful, he managed it and was not guarding against motion as he had.

"I'm not surprised you have back pain Mr. Dorko," said the emergency room doctor. "You have severe arthritic changes back there."

I put my hand on Dad's shoulder, "Those were probably there last week as well," I said.

The doctor looked at me as if I had said something irrelevant.

Dad's fine now. The leg's fine, the back pain was gone after a single day. He speaks of a neighbor now helping out with his sister and he wrote a poem for the nurses at the hospital.

Pain is not just a neurobiologic event and it is not simply a sensation. It has meaning, and it is a perception, thus placing it within each individual's culture, personal history, and recent emotion. My grandmother wasn't around that morning to help my dad as she had so long ago, and that hurt, too.

And my mother? Well, I picked her up to go visit Dad 2 days after his admission. "So," she says in the car, "when did you first hear about your father going to the hospital?"

THE PHOTOGRAPH

I have a photo on my desk of my maternal and paternal grandparents seated beside each other on a couch. It was taken April 15, 1939, my parent's wedding day. It was the only time the four of them were together.

The APTA asked us to celebrate national Physical Therapy Month October 1994 by promoting its version of "good" posture through screenings at selected sites. These include special photos on a grid measuring anatomical alignment and symmetry. There is a list entitled "Tips for Improving Posture" to provide the public.

As the people in my photograph gaze at me, I imagine what kind of conversation the men might have were they to visit one of these screenings.

Therapist: "Well, Mr. Dorko, you certainly hold your head erect, but I see that your left shoulder is a little low and you're not holding your stomach in as it suggests on this list. See right here. It says, 'Don't just wear your stomach muscles, pull them in.'"

Grandpa Dorko replies in a thick Slovak accent: "That shoulder didn't get like this because I was too lazy to hold it up, some lousy unionist hit it with a club when I refused to strike at the coal mine. That mining has something to do with my belly, too. If I hold in my gut I look pretty, but what's left of my lungs can't fill with air. Do you want me to force myself straight and take tiny breaths?"

Therapist: "Well, according to these guidelines, you'd not only look better, but be healthier as well."

Grandpa Dorko: "I felt fine when you took the picture. If I want to look good, I'll put on a new suit. Are you sure I should be holding my shoulder like this? It's beginning to ache."

Therapist: "Yes, well...let's go on to your friend here. Mr. Hinske, your head is well forward of your shoulders and that right leg appears shorter than the other one. Doesn't your neck hurt?"

Grandpa Hinske: "No, never had any pain at all. And that leg, well it was shortened by a bullet during a robbery of my laundry truck 30 years ago. He didn't get the money though, I threw the bag under the truck and..."

Therapist: "Yes, yes, I'm sure it's a good story, but doesn't that awful limp bother you?"

Grandpa Hinske: "Bother me? Why, I never paid it much attention. My grandchildren love the story and the limping never kept me from work. The bullet went clean through and a bandage took care of it. I never tried to hide the limp, it was the least painful way for me to walk."

Therapist: "But don't you think if you held yourself taller and got a lift for your shoe you'd...well, you would look more like this example of good posture sanctioned by the American Physical Therapy Association?" (He holds up a diagram.)

Grandpa Hinske: "Is this supposed to be a person? George, come look at this."

Grandpa Dorko: "Maybe a real skinny one. He's not breathing either."

Therapist: "Look, this is just a kind of generic example. I realize everybody's body is different, but ideally..."

My grandfathers walk away, shaking their heads.

"Imagine telling others to stand up straight for a living," says one.

"They get paid for this?" says the other.

Selected Reading
PT Bulletin. 1994;Jul 27.

THE SCAR

Some men live with an invisible limp, stagger, or drag a leg. Their sons are often angry.
If a man, cautious hides his limp, somebody has to limp it!

Robert Bly, from "My Father's Wedding"

The scar is about 2 inches long and runs vertically along the arch of Joe's right foot.

"What's this scar here?" I ask.

"When I was 11 I was walking barefoot home from playing in the creek and I cut myself real bad. It hurt a lot and I was limping, but knew that if my dad saw what had happened he would whip me. I hid it successfully for about a week, but then he saw that I was still bleeding and in some pain. He didn't beat me because he figured I had already suffered enough."

Joe is now 44 and 5 months ago in a motorcycle accident he suffered a comminuted fracture of the distal fibula and needed an intermedullulary rod to fixate his right tibia as well. He's a steady, hard-working patient and has been getting the best care I have to offer for what seems a long time now. He has recovered from a severe shoulder dislocation followed by an adhesive capsulitis. His x-ray shows excellent healing of the right lower leg and his strength is adequate. But Joe still limps severely and has a good deal of pain at odd times.

When people don't recover as we expect, we can question the adequacy of our care, the motivation of the patient, or even the special circumstances of the event that injured them. But sometimes the fact that our patients don't begin to exist when they are injured or when they first arrive in the waiting room is brought home when we take time to listen to their stories.

When we see scars on the surface of the skin we know at the very least that something foreign has entered there. What entered was not necessarily entirely unwelcomed. Sometimes we look forward to the relief that surgery may offer.

But for the most part the circumstances surrounding the production of a scar are not consciously chosen and can be surrounded by fear, frustration, anger, or helplessness.

Montagu reminds us that the skin and the nervous tissue begin together in the ectoderm and might therefore be considered internal or external manifestations of the same organ. We know that skin irritation elicits sympathetic dominance and a vague but persistent effort to flee or fight will accompany this physiologic state. What happens when we are not allowed to express what is truly in us?

Selzer nearly rhapsodizes when discussing the skin "...it is not the brain nor that heart that is the organ of recollection. It is the skin!...in the crook of his arm she rested the back of her head...this scar upon my cheek that marked the end of love between two brothers. It is all here engraved, that which I was, that which I did..."

Joe hadn't limped since he was 11. It wasn't safe then and now it is. Maybe he's making up for the care he wasn't given. Maybe if therapy can offer him the time and support he needs to touch his deepest scars, the ones we see on the surface will have served a greater purpose.

Selected Reading

Bly R. My father's wedding. *The Man in the Black Coat Turns*. New York, NY: Dial Press; 1981.

Montagu A. *Touching: The Human Significance of the Skin*. New York, NY: Harper & Row; 1968.

Selzer R. *Mortal Lessons: Notes on the Art of Surgery*. New York, NY: Simon & Schuster; 1974.

⊥HE DEFINING MOMENT

Although it hasn't happened recently, I have had patients bring to me photos of their car taken after the crash.

"Can you believe I'm still alive?" they say. "No wonder I still hurt."

This is not usually good news. In my experience, such patients see the incident surrounding their injury as larger than anything since. It has drama, action, and it asks them to play a part. Favorite roles are hero, victim, or martyr.

Of course, a picture isn't necessary. Graphic, repetitive accounts of the events during and immediately after their trauma may be even more powerful in their effect. I once worked with a woman who explained that nearly 20 years earlier a frozen turkey had fallen from the shelf at work and hit her in the knee. Guess who hasn't been right since?

In *The Culture of Pain* by David Morris, the author contends that our current epidemic of chronic pain has its roots in the mid-19th century definition of pain as a purely neurobiologic event. Prior to that, bodily pain was not separated from anguish, sorrow, hunger, depression, or other undesirable human perceptions that were thought to have a deeper meaning, that is, a purpose beyond their presence. Human perception, when examined carefully, informs us about our unique lives and longings, because it is colored by culture, society, theology, economics, and history.

Morris feels that when pain was reduced from a perception to a sensation it lost its meaning. Without meaning very few things are tolerable. Although many of the puzzles about pain have been solved, within its meaning is a mystery that must be explored by each troubled individual. Ultimately, the mysteries of pain are unsolvable, but examining them reveals in bits and pieces the meaning of our lives. Chronic, or perhaps intractable, pain offers an opportunity to the sufferer to pause from "doing" so much and just "being" more. The same is true of illness.

In *The Alchemy of Illness* Kat Duff states, "[In illness] our lives condense, collapse, and recoalesce, requiring changes and we are responsible to those changes. We are not responsible for our illnesses, we are responsible to them, to what they offer and require of all of us, sick and well alike."

Maybe the unconscious is constantly searching for meaning. If we ignore this, it will choose a moment for us to remember and relive until our own mysterious, unique meanings become clear.

If we don't attend carefully to the meaning evident during desirable perception, we may get stuck examining only something like pain, and the unconscious doesn't know that pain is only supposed to be a sensation. It will not be satisfied with attempts to remove it chemically or mechanically. It wants introspection and acceptance. The experience of pain may not make us better, but it should make us more profound.

The moments in life that we choose to define us might be many, and some of us repeat glorious stories. We all hope new moments and meaning are ahead and that we will not be saddled with something tragic or comic (like the flying, frozen turkey).

Patients with chronic pain have such moments. I hope that therapy offers them others, and I know this is more likely when the therapist examines the meaning of their own pain.

Selected Reading
Duff K. *The Alchemy of Illness*. New York, NY: Pantheon; 1993.
Morris D. *The Culture of Pain*. Berkeley, Calif: University of California Press; 1991.

NOTHING'S CHANGED

I read recently of an attorney complaining of pain in his trunk. It began some time after a simple fall from a step ladder while working about his house. Nothing dramatic, no injury, no loss of function.

As it happens, this man, through diligent work and political savvy, had been appointed to a judgeship and, on the surface at least, his personal and professional life was successful and well-ordered.

When the pain persisted and grew, he went to see a family practitioner. As he sat answering questions and submitting to examination, he began to sense that the doctor's office was very much like his courtroom. He felt, however, that now he was in the position of the accused. He knew that although he wanted desperately to ask about the severity of his condition, the doctor/judge was not going to answer. "After all," he reasoned, "I never pronounce sentence before trial, and the rules here are obviously the same."

The pain worsened. Various diagnoses and many forms of medication had virtually no effect on the discomfort and the judge began to find that every aspect of his work and social life was adversely affected. His wife accused him of not carefully following the doctor's orders.

He found that he could obtain considerable relief of his pain at night if he elevated both legs while supine. A young man who worked for him offered to assist with this positioning and the judge was both touched and confused by so thoughtful an act. He never told the doctors that this helped, but his wife did. She said it was no doubt bad for him and the doctor agreed with a smile of "contemptuous affability."

He began to wonder if his pain was in some way connected to the way he had lived his life, but he had always sought to do the "proper" thing and couldn't imagine all his careful posturing and attention to professional duty could possibly have led to so horrible a sensation. In fact, he could not help but feel that his pain was a specific harbinger of his death and this idea scared him most of all.

Throughout this ordeal he spoke to no one of his thoughts; he never expressed the realization that all the truly happy moments of his life ended in early childhood. All he was able to get from his family was pity and, from the doctors, judgmental examinations that proved negative. As he sank into increasing agony, he began to carefully consider that his pain had a special meaning that only he could decipher. It was unique, it was connected to every aspect of his life and it was intractable.

He accepted his pain as part of his life and after a great ordeal of screaming, finally fully expressing his pain, he grew quiet and peaceful. He felt the pain still, but no longer was tormented by its presence. He died very soon afterward.

Many elements of this story are reminiscent of my years dealing with patients whose pain is chronic, undiagnosed, and terribly frustrating to their family and caregivers. Its details and bits of dialogue you can see and hear at any pain clinic in this country, and the basic drama never changes, and the players act out their parts to perfection each day.

The original story is not new, nor does it take place locally. It is "The Death of Ivan Illych" by Leo Tolstoy, and it was written in 1876.

TREATMENT

I treat a lot of patients so I write a great deal about what that is like.

I am very hesitant to write specifically about technique because I feel it implies that I know a great deal more about others' patients than I possibly could. Of course, this hasn't seemed to stop me from writing about what therapists shouldn't do. In this section I speak of the rituals that surround care and the ways we can speak to our patients that are meaningful and revealing.

My personal tendency as a therapist is to allow patients to express their health in a painless and unconsciously motivated fashion. This requires not so much that they trust me, but rather that I trust them.

PAIN AND EXPRESSION

Before I begin any lecture, I notice that I pass through a ritual of movement that has not varied much over the years. I draw myself straight, I expand my shoulders, and I try to fill my face with an expression that is both intelligent and sincere. In short, I strike a pose. The dictionary says I "pretend to be something I am not."

My audience never objects. We live in a society where striking poses is the norm. To move spontaneously and authentically is to invite disapproval. People would stare, they would wonder what was wrong with you and, if they couldn't stop you in some way, they would turn their attention elsewhere. I don't think I'm exaggerating here. Just try a little self-expression through movement in public and see what happens. It will probably work in front of your family as well.

Of course, in our culture, verbal expression is permitted, even honored. The more a person authentically and spontaneously speaks, the more they are encouraged by many of our institutions to advance, to ascend.

I understand that in China the converse is true. While verbal expression is carefully chosen and monitored for its political correctness, the parks each morning are filled with individuals doing tai chi. Al Huang explains that tai chi is not really a series of movements or poses, but a physical expression of what the unconscious desires. He says, "true dancing is letting your awareness flow into movement."

Physical and emotional pain are difficult to separate. David Morris says they are like two hands clasped together. But it seems clear to me that when we speak of our emotional pain, it is eased, and when we speak of our physical pain it is not. We know too, that the verbal expression that eases emotional pain cannot be scripted.

Would it follow that movement must be equally spontaneous if it were to relieve physical pain? Does this explain why choreographed regimes of exercise often don't reduce pain in significant or prolonged ways? Is the epidemic of chronic physical pain in our society in some way the result of our cultural posturing, posing, and distaste for personal physical expression?

If I don't say what I want to, my throat tightens. This is simply the isometric contraction of muscles that give voice to my thoughts once I permit verbal expression. Only then will the muscles relax. I wonder sometimes if the skeletal muscle tightness we see in patients with pain isn't a similar process in the periphery, a process only completed once spontaneous movement is promoted. I tell my patients that the tightness they feel is movement unrequited, and they find it's true.

When I pose before a lecture, I am playing the part I've chosen in my culture. Maybe my escape (so far) from chronic pain is the result of my tendency to honor and express my unconsciously motivated desire to move whenever I can. This is something my culture does not like.

I practiced a long time before I understood this and used such thinking to help myself and my patients. The time was spent working to see my own posing for what is was, and for what it did to me. As Bertrand Russell put it: "We do not know who discovered water, but we can be certain that it wasn't a fish."

Selected Reading

Huang A. *Embrace Tiger, Return to Mountain—The Essence of T'ai Chi*. Moab, Utah: Real People Press; 1973.

Morris D. *The Culture of Pain*. Berkeley, Calif: University of California Press; 1991.

MOVEMENT AND DESIRE

To be nobody-but-yourself in a world which is doing its best, night and day, to make you everybody else—means to fight the hardest battle which any human being can fight; and never stop fighting

e.e. cummings

In my essay "Origins" I emphasized that mechanical deformation was the origin of most of the pain we might help with physical means.

I consider this a deceptively simple idea because it makes no mention of why movement hurts at some times and not at others, or how a comfortable, static position can become painful.

What I didn't mention was the element of adaptive potential. This quality of autonomic flow and balance determines how much deformation is possible without pain. For me, a large adaptive potential is displayed by competitive swimmers. Their fluid tone allows them to painlessly tolerate repetitive, forceful, prolonged, and acute deformation. My patients are usually at the other end of the autonomic spectrum.

Simply put, sympathetic dominance decreases our tolerance for mechanical tension and parasympathetic dominance increases it.

Much of what we call physical therapy boils down to finding the movement that both decreases mechanical tension and sympathetic tone. It is clear that the primary tissue capable of changing us autonomically in this way is the nervous tissue itself.

For a long time now I've been convinced that for all my attempts to sense dysfunction through means of examination, I still can't tell a patient which movement will take them out of the twist they've uniquely acquired. One day I simply stopped coercing them manually and discovered this: Everybody is unconsciously attempting to reduce their neural tension by means both subtle and obvious. This attempt to move is concurrent with life, but ordinarily we have no sense of it, do not fully express it, and are typically taught to distrust it. The movement may contain a rhythmic quality at times, but other than that it is wholly characterized by its effortlessness and spontaneity.

This movement is least likely to be expressed in situations where we tend to pose, posture, or feel concerned about the judgment of others. In other words, just about everywhere.

The movement needed to reduce neural tension is the expression of desire. That is, it comes from each of us uniquely, personally, and intensely. It can't be taught or choreographed because it is instinctive, primal, and unpredictable. It is done in an effort to please no one but yourself.

Our culture does not encourage the authentic expression of unconscious desire outside the institutions of art, and there it is only tolerated among those with a "gift."

All that most of my patients really need to do is what they want to do. If I can somehow give them an environment that makes it safe to express that, they soften and feel much better.

The real struggle begins when they walk out the door and face a culture that demands something else.

<u>Suggested Reading</u>
Dorko BL. Adaptive potential: a new concept in pain of mechanical origin. *PT Forum.* 1988;7(29).

HOPE AND DIAPHRAGMATIC BREATHING

Often I feel I am engaged in an epic struggle with my own culture.

I realize that that is a very dramatic statement, but I should also say that there is no evidence that my culture is in any way aware of my striving against it. This is a pitifully one-sided battle and I am doomed. It's like the culture is an Acme rocket launcher and I am Wile E. Coyote.

The title of this essay contains two very familiar but remarkably disparate elements. Like a surrealistic painting of melting watches, it grasps your attention because these things aren't supposed to go together. But the feeling of hope and the action of the diaphragm are connected by cultural imperatives so powerful as to color feeling and activity each day, each to the detriment of our patients.

Let me explain.

Have you ever explained to a patient what his or her problem is and predict recovery consequent to care and exercise only to hear the patient say, "I hope you're right." Better yet, a patient returns to your office obviously improved. After you point out how much better he or she is doing, the patient says, "I hope so."

I don't know about you, but I find such statements absolutely chilling. When I hear them I sense that the patient will never significantly improve, or if he or she does, the patient won't notice it.

I know that we are specifically taught that hope is a positive, if not essential, quality for life itself, but to hope is to live in some imagined future, and it specifically gives us the same message over and over. The message is: "The current situation is unacceptable, it is not good enough."

Such a feeling is disastrous for change precisely because knowledge and acceptance are essential for change to begin. Hoping, while honored in society as a desirable attribute, stands in the way of understanding what we currently have, gifts included.

I don't want my patients to hope. I want them to notice what they can do at this moment and I want them to understand how their condition will most likely change favorably if they attend to their current functioning.

Now let's turn to one of my favorite modalities: diaphragmatic breathing.

I can't think of any single bodily activity that promotes health as surely or persistently as regular, complete, powerful movement of the diaphragm. The medical literature agrees wholeheartedly. (I have the references in case anyone is interested.)

Yet I rarely see patients breathing this way and, in fact, most therapists don't. Believe me, I've seen hundreds of PTs at workshops in the past 20 years, and even demonstrating a single, deep diaphragmatic breath is a struggle for the majority.

Thoracic ventilation leads to increased sympathetic tone, unnecessary muscle tone, anxiety, and pain. Why don't we as therapists work to reduce it in ourselves and others?

Let me ask you this: Do the models in the magazines ever let their abdominal wall expand? Does the model of "correct" posture on the wall of your clinic display an abdomen with the fullness of inhalation or the flatness possible only when we either exhale or "hold in our gut?"

The culture encourages us to hope, thus the gifts of the present moment along with true understanding are lost. The culture tells us that breathing like Pavarotti will make us look fat. And surely we don't want that.

Both of these directives are untrue. Maybe therapy can turn the tide toward health and awareness with less hope, more understanding, and a deep breath.

<u>Suggested Reading</u>
Pema C. Abandon any hope of fruition. *Pilgrimage*. 1994;20(2).

BABY BEAR'S BED

"She came finally to a small bed and laid down upon it. It was not too hard, and not too soft. It was just right. Very soon she fell fast asleep."

From "Goldilocks and the Three Bears"

I don't often write of the specifics of technique. I'm convinced what we do should naturally follow a model of the body that we can explain and defend.

It follows that your model's reaction to provocation would be a function of its make-up down to the cellular level. The qualities you assign to the tissues must be confirmed by adequate research. Without that, justifying technique by shrugging your shoulders and saying, "Hey, it works," is probably not a good idea. Especially if you are standing near me.

I've long held a specific aversion to heavy pressure with the knuckles on tender body parts. The efficacy of this treatment must take a back seat to its rationale, especially since it is commonly painful. While defending this technique, although it seems to provide only a temporarily analgesia, a sports medicine therapist told me that her athletes need "quick results." I guess she thinks my factory workers, teachers, secretaries, and accountants are satisfied with less.

The many techniques that comprise manual care are notorious for providing analgesia alone. If we don't effectively promote correction and a return to normal autonomic tone with our handling, well, that's just not good enough.

Manual care that leads to correction and prolonged relief may come from many theoretical directions, but there is probably an aspect of its force that is common to all forms; it is enough to inform the body of its intent without being perceived as potentially harmful.

When I demonstrate technique at a workshop, the location and direction of my force is easily described, but the students struggle with the degree of force used because it changes so frequently.

O. Fred Donaldson speaks eloquently of touch in play therapy. "The skin becomes a barrier if touch is undertaken too harshly, and aside from the obvious, there are many subtle forms of intrusive touch."

The force necessary to elicit self-correction (the type of manual care I personally employ) is not a constant, and it can be difficult to predict or describe. I am always searching for a response to pressure that includes unconscious motivation, warmth, and effortlessness. As long as these qualities grow, I'll stay where I am and I'll adjust the direction and amplitude of my pressure as the patient dictates.

Ultimately I am seeking repose, but only as the end result of unique movement. My touch implies that. And from moment to moment, it changes with the patient. My patients taught me this. I don't think you can learn it at a workshop.

Whoever built Baby Bear's bed created something Goldilocks simply couldn't resist. Sometimes therapy can provide a similar touch for those who need the rest.

Selected Reading
Donaldson OF. *Playing By Heart*. Deerfield Beach, Fla: Health Communications Inc; 1993.

THE VASE

Imagine that one day you are handed a vase and told that is now your job to hold it with your hands alone. You cannot put it down or give it to somebody else. You don't own it, but it is your responsibility to keep it with you and this is what you are paid to do.

I am often given credit for having remarkably sensitive hands. Therapists watching me work speak wistfully of how wonderful it must be to have such a gift. If they don't think it's genetically acquired, they assume my sensitivity is the result of years of concentrated effort.

I don't buy any of this. If either were true, I think I would know it.

Imagine now that you've been holding on to the vase for a few minutes and that you are told from a perfectly reliable source that the vase is worth millions of dollars.

How might you change? I've asked many therapists this very questions and they almost always insist that they be allowed to put the vase down despite my specific admonition to the contrary. In time, they may describe their hands in relation to the vase now that they have this new knowledge.

Assuming that its worth might mean it is fragile, their hands now grasp it more fully, but gripping is out. In their imagination they become increasingly aware of the vase's shape and tendency to respond to gravity as they shift its weight.

If I prod them a bit, they tell me that something worth this much might be interesting to see. They look at it carefully. Its texture, glaze, and shape might reveal why it is so expensive, and the therapists usually wish they knew more about vases.

In short, there is no distinct increase in the sensitivity of the therapist. All the sensitivity they use in the end was with them when first handed the vase. It is much more accurate to say that they now appreciate what it is they are holding. Their gentle handling and interest in the subtleties of the vase follow what they know it is worth. Before that, care and attention to the holding was haphazard at best.

Although we don't ordinarily assign monetary worth to the human body, something akin to that is evident in all contact with others. The potential referral source (read: money in the bank) is more likely to elicit more interest and consideration from us than some of the patients he or she sends. This is the nature of business, like it or not.

I feel that the role of the physical therapist should include an appreciation of the body that is reflected in the way we hold it. But what is our reputation? Most patients come to me fearful of being poked, prodded, and painfully bent. It's what their friends got for similar conditions and I can understand their fear.

It is absolutely impossible to handle another with care and wonder without feeling you deserve the same. When I was handed this "vase" years ago, I wanted to put it down too. I felt not up to the task and my methods reflected that. I was known to relinquish this responsibility to an aide or assistant, a protocol or machine. This doesn't always work very well, and it added nothing to my appreciation for the patient or myself.

My hands are not unusually sensitive, nor are my skills especially difficult to acquire. But when I'm with others on the job, I can sense their worth, and I hold them with care.

PLAYING HOCKEY

When I was 8 years old my Aunt Alice gave our family a table hockey game. The players moved in slots on the ice and were manipulated by rods that could be pushed, pulled, or twisted at either end of the rink.

This was easily the most popular gift we ever got and my brothers and sisters and I spent hours whacking a tiny puck with little metal hockey players. Their movements were confined to straight lines and tight circles, at first difficult to connect with our flailing hands. Eventually the hand and the rod and the player were synchronized in our heads and we learned to pass and defend and react with remarkable speed. The movement of the players was accurate and efficient if somewhat jerky and prone to sudden spins. In fact, I personally still skate that way to this day.

Compared to today's video games, this was not only low-tech but required relatively gross motor skills. But you could really feel it when you played. Body English actually made a difference if you used enough to tip the rink. The game produced vibrations in your hands that were eventually visceral in effect. You learn or solve a video game. This game you felt.

I remember keeping score I suppose, but mainly I remember being lost in the activity along with my siblings. O. Fred Donaldson writes of the essence of play in childhood: "[Play is] trust...in a web of relationships of which one is part." He insists that the adult imposition of "contest" upon the play of the child restricts the spontaneity essential for the growth it may produce. "Winning and playing are not only different behaviors, but different views of the world." In translating play as contest, we have given the labels, definitions, and relationships of one form of behavior to another without recognizing that they are significantly different concepts and forms of behavior," and "Play is not a matter of effort but of grace. In play there is only one side."

I remember watching Berta Bobath "play" with a parietic limb. It was a re-entry into the innocent, nonjudgmental exploration of the child that she wanted to elicit as she displayed it herself. This was so remarkably different from the gross manipulation, the wrestling match of some other forms of care I'd seen.

In his classic *Zen in the Art of Archery*, Herrigel is struggling with his release of the bowstring. He is told: "Grasp the bowstring as the child grasps the proffered finger." Once he finds the faith to do this he can find the courage necessary to release it effortlessly. He plays with his immediate environment and thus gathers trust and awareness. I think that many clinicians can relate to that sort of attitude when they relate and blend well with any patient.

Well, my brother gave my son Alex a hockey game for Christmas. Plastic this time, but otherwise the same. As we play I can feel the old familiar patterns in me rising to the surface. Of course, at my age they don't rise to the surface as quickly as they do in my 7-year-old, so he often thinks that he wins. He doesn't yet know that he can't win unless I lose. And since I'm only "playing," I can't. I spoke to him about all this and he asked me if I would feel the same if I weren't a PT. That's a good question.

Selected Reading
Donaldson OF. Play to win and every victory is a funeral. *Somatics*. 1984;4(4).
Herrigel E. *Zen in the Art of Archery*. New York, NY: Vintage Books; 1971.

Suggested Reading
Donaldson OF. Chrysanthemum swords: towards an understanding of play as a universal martial art. *Somatics*. 1985-1986;5(3).

Jt's TIME FOR "CLINICAL IMPROVEMENT"

"Hello, and welcome to 'Clinical Improvement,' the show that spotlights physical therapy and the machines that make it work. I'm your host and director of the fully equipped office you see behind me. As always, I will be assisted by my staff therapist, Harley.

"Today, we're going to consider the many ways we can attack a patient with low back pain."

"Uh, excuse me, sir, but don't you think we ought to first address the issue of pertinent history and assessment in so vague a complaint?"

"What for? We have the diagnosis right here on the referral: 'low back pain.' What are you trying to do, upset the doctor? Listen, I know this guy and he's good for five referrals a week as long as we don't examine the patients. Anyway, if we want to figure out what is wrong we can just hook his back to this Binford Hyperstim Reflexometer. Two or three maneuvers and his entire muscular function is displayed on this graph. Look, there's the problem right there."

"How do you know that that pattern of muscular function is not present to protect and possibly even correct the underlying deformation in the patient's neural tissue? Here's a study published in the APTA Journal indicating that there's no correlation between muscular strength and joint position."

"Harley, do you know how much this machine costs? Let's move on to the treatment. I like to begin back pain with a few minutes on the Binford Neuromuscular Electromatic Mobilizer. You can crank this baby up to 500 volts while simultaneously delivering a 50 pound per square inch blow to the transverse processes at three different levels."

"Does this guy hurt for lack of electrical stimulation? Do all the levels of his spinal column have the same restriction?"

"Look Harley, I'm talking about charging for two modalities at once here and I don't even have to be in the room. Just by flipping the switch I can add a heating element that will pay for your next continuing ed course, so watch it. I can see what you're getting at though. You think I don't get in there and handle these people enough. Well, I have just the thing for that right here. You see these gloves? They are attached to the new Binford Multi-Channel Isotoner Manual Massago-Master. With these I can give this guy some manual therapy he will never forget. You want individualized care? Look right here, 'One size fits all.' Even that puny aide can deliver a wallop with these babies."

"You seem to be advocating the use of more force or stimulation every time a problem doesn't resolve with simple rest and medication. Don't you think we ought to consider what the patients themselves might contribute to correction? How can the patients ever understand that their pain is the end result of a process and not an event, that it is the result of the way that they are and not something they possess that you are supposed to somehow take away? They think treatment is over when the bell goes off on the machine and they take nothing with them."

"Harley, maybe you should have your own show. You can call it 'The Wimpo Therapy Hour.' You're going to have a lot of trouble finding a sponsor, though. Well folks, that's all we have time for today. Tune in next week when we introduce the new Binford Traction Master and Musculotenderizer. It's awesome."

SEDUCTION

I sat at a meeting of people seeking a cure recently. There were men and women of all ages and styles of dress. In the group of about 20, I counted five wigs.

I really do not want to go into details but basically this was a gathering of people who wanted to learn about the use and marketing of magnets that were supposed to relieve pain. According to the speakers (qualifications unknown), the magnets worked by stirring up the blood flow with an alternating polarity. Just exactly why this would relieve pain I cannot say. I felt it was best not to ask.

The majority of the meeting was consumed by marketing information. I could have gotten pillows and a mattress pad and slept in a marvelous magnetic field. I could sell this stuff and make fabulous profits.

I escaped.

I suppose a lot could be written about the holes in this theory of pain relief. What fascinated me though, was the way I felt when I heard the testimonials about successful application. A part of me wanted to believe that something as simple as this would help my patients. I heard a voice saying, "What could it hurt? It's harmless, and you've got a few people you sure aren't helping any other way." (I know many physicians feel the same way about physical therapy.)

I have been through this sort of thing before. Heck, a few years ago I was actually hanging some people by their ankles. You would think that I would eventually realize that placebo is like a honeymoon—it's great, but it can't last. In 20 years I have yet to find anything really simple and easy that resolves otherwise intractable problems. The body seems to defy simple solutions by virtue of its inherent complexity and unpredictability.

Still, caregivers are easily seduced by radical ideas accompanied by stories of success. We have a stake in helping others and there is always that little voice asking, "What could it hurt?"

Perhaps it would be best if we considered what these stories of success tell us about human disability. It seems that people can be sick in two basic ways. This was noticed in an observation by George

Bernard Shaw while at the grotto in Lourdes. Seeing the cave walls lined with no longer needed aides he remarked, "All those canes and crutches and braces; no wigs, no glass eyes, no artificial limbs."

SANTA AND ME

"You can't always get what you want."

Mick Jagger

About this time each year I have a little talk with Santa. It's a wide ranging discussion and not always confined to the personal desires of my family and how we might devise a payment plan extending well into the new year.

This year we got onto the subject of needs and wants. He said, "I see it this way—needs are the things we can buy, and wants are the things unattainable in my workshop, or even in the mall. The problem with Christmas is this: people think they can buy the things they want, but money only provides needs. They want things like peace, love, respect, admiration, and health, but I can only provide things like sweaters, jewelry, and Nintendo. Often by noon Christmas day, people feel kind of empty because their Christmas list was mislabeled. It said 'I want' and it should have said 'I need'."

"Wait a minute," I said. "Did I hear you say that health was something I couldn't buy?"

"Of course it isn't. Now I know that health care has a price, but all the money in the world isn't going to provide you with a certain metabolism or the behaviors necessary to maintain or improve your body's functions. You can buy a treadmill (he shows me a picture) but running on it is another matter."

"But what about all those ads from the health clubs showing the picture of a great body with the cost of membership next to it? What about the money people pay me for treatment? Don't those dollars buy some health?"

"No," he shook his beard. "That money pays for care, for attention, for information, and for time near an expert. People carry their health with them. They pay you to help them reveal it. What they eventually have they earn through discipline and self-acceptance. I understand that genetics are important here, too, but I don't worry about that. My job is to know whether you've been bad or good."

"I think I'm beginning to see why my stationary bicycle has never helped me and why all the books I buy teach me so much. I actually read the books," I said.

"If more people understood that," Santa replied, "it would certainly make my job a lot easier. I swear, if I have to deliver one more Salad Shooter..."

"You know, Santa," I continued, "what you've said has very large implications for physical therapy if not health care in general. I think the new national hea..."

Santa's cheeks began to grow even redder than usual. I was concerned: "Are you all right, Santa?"

"Yes, yes, but I think we'll have to continue this discussion next year. Right now, Barrett, you just gotta get off my lap."

*I*N THE NIGHT

I was an orderly in a physical therapy department at the age of 16. This was a good job for a number of reasons, not the least of which was that I never had to work weekends. In fact, therapy was not provided on weekends in most places with any regularity until I was in practice a few years.

I graduated from school during the golden age of modalities. We were taught that primary problems of pain should be treated as if they were always concurrent with tissue injury, and my job was to promote healing by drawing blood to the painful part. I didn't need skill so much as I needed electrical outlets.

Anyway, I entered practice having been given two distinct messages: real pain and injury were always concurrent and therapy was provided only during weekdays after sun-up.

Once in practice, I was soon faced with two new facts: significant tissue damage was commonly absent in chronic pain and people often needed therapy when darkness fell. In fact, night was the worst time for many of my patients and it remains so today.

Karen Fiser, in a wheelchair and chronically in pain, has expressed her ordeal in an amazing book of poetry entitled *Words Like Fate and Pain.* In "Night Shift," she writes in part:

> *At first*
> *it is the same nightmare:*
> *the pain factory*
> *deep in the interior,*
> *the blast furnace going*
> *half the night,*
> *driving the muffled*
> *engines to make enough*
> *hurt.*

How many times have you heard, "I wish you could have seen me about 3:00 a.m. this morning!"?

Fiser's poem graphically describes the rise in sympathetic tone that peaks by 4:00 a.m. (half the night) and is present in all of us. As I grow colder, another blanket will help, but those with irritated nervous tissue lose the adaptive potential that makes sleep possible at 11:00 p.m. Now they are faced with pain that defies a simple change in position. They have to shift their physiology and this means they have to get up and move. They wonder: What have I done wrong? Which way can I lie comfortably? Is it time for another pill? They wish the therapist could see them now.

What would my practice be like if I began seeing patients at 11:00 p.m.? I think that the same people I see in the daylight, with their comments on the weather, their jobs, or the traffic, would speak of issues more personal and closely connected to their pain. The unconscious normally rules at night and if I want instinctive movement and less posing from my patient, I will probably find it easily at 2:00 a.m.

Karen Fiser may not know why pain often increases at night. I would guess no one has told her of the relation between physiologic state and nociceptive firing. But she knows that the night offers a time to change that is more profound than anything that happens in the glare of the clinic's light. In the final verse she states this starkly:

Like the night animal tearing
in the teeth of pain
machinery, you will not
get out of this the same

Maybe if therapists understood as much about the night and what a dangerous opportunity it offers, we could help more during the daylight.

Selected Reading

Fiser K. *Words Like Fate and Pain*. Cambridge, Mass: Zoland Books; 1992.

Gellhorn E. *Somatic-Automatic Integrations: Physiologic Basis and Clinical Implications*. Minneapolis, Minn: University of Minnesota Press; 1967.

PAIN AND POETICS

Often in therapy we wrestle with intractable pain, that is, pain whose cause cannot be found or, if found, cannot be removed. Of course, this definition implies that to some extent the caregiver decides whether or not the patient's pain is intractable. When faced with such a situation, protocols, goal-setting, team meetings, and sophisticated functional assessments may not be as helpful as simply bearing witness with some depth of understanding and physiological insight.

In *Migraine*, Oliver Sacks states, "Migraine is a remarkably primitive reaction involving massive alterations of vegetative activity and behavior." This description links the pain of a migrainous episode to instinct, for humans as well as all other mammals. Although it is not possible to say that animals have migraines, the behavior they exhibit in times of stress mirrors the migraine patient's withdrawal from the world.

I'll get back to that, but I want to shift to something else.

The Welsh poet David Whyte wrote a series of poems related to his prolonged periods of silent meditation. He begins "Imagine My Surprise":

Imagine my surprise,
sitting a full hour
in silent and irremediable
fear of the world

Having felt this same fear in times of silence, I immediately relate to his words. Sacks points out that the mammalian reaction to the instinct of fear is two-fold, although the acute phase (flight or fight, sensory vigilance, and the emotional correlates of rage or terror) is usually the only one mentioned. Of equal importance is the physiologic and behavioral response to chronic fear (i.e., pallor, sweat, prostration, withdrawal, and immobilization). The emotional correlates are not described, but it is generally accepted that as fear spreads from the diencephalon through the human cortex, it may be mutated to a variety of emotions, or no emotion at all.

Whyte's poem goes on:

to find the body
forgetting
it's own fear the instant

it opened and placed
its unassuming hands
on life's enduring pain

As the migraine sufferer withdraws, in fact, behaves as if irresistibly attacked, they create an opportunity for introspection, interoception (body awareness), and instinctive reactions unencumbered by human emotion.

Perhaps they inwardly place their "unassuming hands" on their own fear. This ritual is usually very effective.

Pain once considered intractable is entirely relieved and the patient often feels a surge of energy, the body completely reanimated. Maybe the underlying processes responsible for the attack are markedly diminished and difficult to reproduce, maybe not.

Whyte completes the poem:

and the world for one
moment
closed its terrifying eyes
in gratitude
Saying
"This is my body, I am found."

Sometimes therapy helps those with intractable pain in a way that is like reciting this poem with the verses reversed. Give it a try.

Selected Reading
Sacks O. *Migraine*. Berkeley, Calif: University of California Press.
Whyte D. *The Poetry of David Whyte*. Langly, Wash: Many Rivers Press.

Suggested Reading
Dorko BL. *The suppression of flight*.

A PRACTICE MADE BY HAND

I have a rocking chair in my waiting room that my sister Laurel found at an antique store.

Over a 150 years ago somebody formed its broad, comfortable seat on short legs, and from a single piece of wood carved two opposing dragons, teeth bared and leaping across the backrest. Anyone seated in this chair is simultaneously accepted completely by the seat, while his or her head rests between two remarkably fierce images that are mythical, slightly asymmetric, and beautiful.

Estes suggests that we can pursue a "hand-made life" and when I read this I was immediately drawn to it. She says such a life would proceed from a clear vision of its unfolding and that it would be lived slowly, but surely. Offers of faster or easier ways of moving along its path are discarded if they do not include the unique piecing together of our inner and outer lives. Such a life is characterized by small, faithful acts performed thoughtfully with an eye on what we want to create. Only after a long time is the whole of such a life evident to others.

Perhaps such a life could be just a part of the world we move in. It is certainly hard in the world today to remain thoughtful, faithful, and simple in all that we do. The culture we live in moves so fast that if we can just avoid being trampled we may still be left behind. I want to talk about the possibility of a hand-made practice.

As I watch corporations devour the independent practitioners I've known for years, I feel that my own business may go the way of the stegosaurus. As long as the managed care industry is convinced that physical therapy is akin to pharmacy and is easily reduced to generic prescriptions, we are all fair game. We know what the trends are and a place for the care we would like to provide may not be part of the future medical system.

The chair in my waiting room sits among several others that look like they will last a few more years, but I know that since they are upholstered, repairs will be necessary soon. There is nothing replaceable about the rocker and, in fact, it gets less use because it's low and my patients with backache know better than to use it. By its nature it is used sparingly and it endures. I've seen patients inspect it carefully and many want to take it home.

In an effort to build a practice than endures I provide a kind of care that is very dependent on my personality and unique perception of the body. This cannot be stamped out on a form and so far I've not seen it duplicated. I try not to judge my patients just because their problems are chronic or the possibility exists that their pain provides secondary gains. I think this is universally true. I don't have a "back program" and diagnoses do not automatically evoke a protocol of care. I am willing to take the time to let the patient reveal his or her health, much in the same way that carver let the rocker reveal its dragons.

Such a practice can't afford full-page advertising in the Yellow Pages. It is not understood or even preferred by the medical community, and nobody wants to buy it and finance my retirement. But my patients like it, and, as with this essay, I do the work myself—by hand.

Selected Reading
Estes. *Sounds True Catalogue.* 1993;Feb.

$\mathcal{T}$HE ORPHAN

"This started to really bother me 4 months ago, but I waited to come in."

The speaker is a patient I saw 2 years earlier for a similar complaint of pain. She did very well with a brief series of visits and used her new-found body awareness and exercises to prevent more trouble for a while afterward. Then, understandably, she began to equate the absence of pain with the presence of health, so she stopped attending to her way of being once again. Now her body is screaming for attention and she has returned for help.

This 4-month delay used to be the kind of thing that really bothered me. I adhered to the notion that chronic pain necessarily required more care. I no longer think so. I used to think that people did not trust me to help them. This was not true. I used to feel frustrated at the return of an old complaint. Now I remember that it is money in the bank.

Still, the hesitance to pursue care until there has been an inordinate amount of suffering is so common that I often wonder about it.

My courses, populated by therapists, are no exception. Many students admit that they have chronically recurrent problems for which they do not seek care. On top of this, the care they give to patients with similar symptoms is mistrusted and they won't "waste their time" having these things done to them. They forge ahead, ever the caregiver, never the caretaker.

My personal fascination with archetypal psychology makes a book by Carol Pearson one of my favorites. It is *Awakening the Heroes Within*. It is about the many beings that metaphorically live within us and drive our vast array of behaviors and reactions. As a general rule each of the archetypes must have a way of clearly expressing itself or it will emerge unexpectedly in an immature of "shadow" form.

The archetype of the Orphan is especially relevant to this discussion. The Orphan is that part of us that feels the pain of betrayal, the inevitable loneliness of at least some parts of life, and the helplessness that illness can produce. To deny that we have at times felt this way is to reject the Orphan's gifts of empathy, a tendency to work with others and, most importantly, the ability to ask for help when we need it.

The Orphan denied often makes us whiny or needy without the will to move actively toward appropriate help. Two years ago I worked for 10 days while developing pneumonia. Rather than stop when I should have, I ended up in the hospital, a trip my Orphan might have saved me.

When my patients do not care for themselves and then delay going for help, I think of how weak their Orphan may be. Perhaps the therapists who complain but do not get treatment fear the helplessness that sickness and care imply and they want to maintain control. Maybe that is why they became therapists.

In the 13th century Rumi (1207-1273) wrote a poem about the Orphan:

Do you think I know what I'm doing?
That for one breath of half-breath I belong to myself?
As much as a pen knows what it's writing
Or the ball can guess where it's going next.

I give it to my patients, and to myself.

Selected Reading

Moyne J, Barks C. *Open Secret—Versions of Rumi.* Putney, Vt: Threshold Books; 1984.
Pearson C. *Awakening the Heroes Within.* New York, NY: Harper Collins; 1991.

WHEN THE HERO RESTS

In 1980 my daughter Jennie was 1 year old. When I came home from work I would hold her in my right arm for a while. Each time she would reach for the pen in my shirt pocket, lift it carefully, and place it in my hand. It was a game she only played with me, and now that I think about it, I really miss it.

I attend several conferences each year and listen to others speak of their methods of management for pain. These speeches rarely affect my own practice and sometimes I worry that I've grown blind to problems that another therapist would see and correct. On the other hand, at least I don't race from one technique to another like I once did.

Listening to others I gain more insight into how and why I often see things so differently, and why my form of handling is rarely used elsewhere.

The underlying theme of care for pain in most clinics these days is control and aggression. In one manner or another the patient is taught to control posture, movement, behavior, diet, painful expressions, undesirable muscular activity, and hopefully, pain. This control is achieved through an aggressive routine of exercise designed to recondition the body.

The therapist's role is to control the previously mentioned aspects of the patient's life through instruction, manual coercion, verbal exhortation, and by ignoring or overtly disapproving of behaviors they feel will retard recovery. This is work best done by a kind of warrior/therapist personally willing to aggressively pursue health through effort and self-denial. Appearance and strength mean a great deal to them.

I should say that I know programs of this sort are often successful for patients and that the therapists in charge are bright, dedicated, and often represent the best our profession has to offer.

If I have a problem with this method of care it is not because of what it offers, but because of what it omits and implies.

The heroic tradition of recovery from disability is deeply rooted in our culture. From "The Best Years of Our Lives" to the recent stories about the NFL's Dennis Byrd, the mass media has lionized effort, willful control, and aggressive elimination of our weaker tendencies. It is no wonder physical therapists seek a prominent role here.

But sometimes it is clear that a more thoughtful, sensitive part of ourselves, a part not strong or attractive, leads us out of trouble. These are personal attributes most likely to appear at quiet moments when effort and judgment and goals and expectations do not surround us. A gym full of weights and lists of repetitions do not encourage unique personal expression through movement. If that is what a patient needs, they will not recover there and more than likely will be chastised for a lack of effort.

Writing for publication can be a difficult, lonely, foolish, simple, scary, exciting, and exhilarating task. Recovery from pain has many of the same qualities and I'm not certain that only a hero can lead every patient through this.

Today I held my partner's daughter, Alexis, in my arm after I arrived at work. She's not heroic, but tiny, frail, accepting, and fully present with everything around her. She will turn 1 year old in a couple of weeks. She reached into my pocket, removed the pen, and placed it in my hand.

Ritual

In the movie "The Big Chill" I remember watching Kevin Kline gently place the stylus of a record player on a record and wait anxiously, perfectly still, for the first few notes. At their arrival he is changed in his body right from the very center. His face is transformed.

Those of us old enough to remember music before audio cassettes and CDs are very familiar with the ritual surrounding the playing of records. It began with gazing at the album cover and then carefully handling its contents by the edges only, fingers spread, no gripping. Vision came into play as the record was inspected and perhaps even blown upon (dryly, of course). Placement of the record on the turntable and the needle on the record required slow, patient movement and was accompanied by perfectly coordinated vision and breathing. You couldn't talk and do this well at the same time. I had friends who took much better care of their albums than anything else in their lives. For this they were rewarded with high quality sound and a collection they treasured. I don't know anybody who treasures their tape collection this way.

Rituals contain a few simple elements available to all of us. There is first of all movement. More specifically, a movement of the body that requires it to leave what it is doing otherwise and attend to this task so that its feeling is deepened. This seems to connect us with something else, something universally common. Finally, ritual uses very few words.

Robert Johnson points out that ritual can be remarkably effective in the resolution of conflict within the unconscious. This is because the unconscious doesn't know the difference between a ritual act and an actual act. Once we decide that one thing symbolizes another and we treat the symbol as needed there is a movement toward resolution that will be reflected favorably in the physical body as well. Simply put, the conflict within seeks order and if this is not done consciously it will simply be done unconsciously, often neurotically. That is, the world around us begins to represent the enemy within and we see it as dangerous and untrustworthy.

When we become a participant in a ritual that addresses our needs, we literally feel better. Usually this happens accidentally, but sometimes we go to a place where we can move in a thoughtful way, and in a way that deepens our sense of self, where we are supported and few words are used.

I feel certain that effective therapy includes the elements of ritual, but often that part of our care is accidental and given little credit for its power. When we institute new procedures because some research indicates they will "work" better than the old ones some questions come to mind. How did the old procedure ever work at all? Was it the ritual? Will the new procedure allow us time for a similar ritual?

I don't mean to say that effective care isn't possible without thoughtful movement, attention to detail, and nonverbal communication. But these elements shouldn't be ignored and they might be mainly what the patient needs.

When pain persists and its origins are not entirely visible, the presence of some internal conflict must be considered. Ritual may work to resolve something no machine can measure or ablate.

Selected Reading

Johnson R. *Owning Your Own Shadow*. San Francisco, Calif: Harper Collins; 1991.
Ventura M. Possibilities of ritual. *LA Weekly*. 1992;Jan 17.

Suggested Reading

Dorko BL. *The suppression of flight*.

DON'T RELAX

"For living things, all restlessness is directed towards the achievement of tranquility."

Jonathan Miller

"Well, I must admit that I spent a lot of time swinging a pickax yesterday. I got rid of some roots so the lilies could come up next spring."

Mary is explaining why her shoulders still hurt despite my best efforts in the office last week. The comment doesn't surprise me. Mary warned me that she had always been a "doer."

"I've never been one to just sit around. I have a sister like that though." (It doesn't sound like a compliment.)

Mary's diagnosis of degenerative joint disease isn't surprising. She's 68 years old, and I can easily visualize the x-rays. It's picturing this tiny woman with a pickax that I have trouble with. I asked her if she had used a sledgehammer much during the past year.

"Sure."

Most of the time such a patient would be directed to rest and relax, to stop doing anything forceful with his or her arms for awhile at least. But since Mary's onset of pain was insidious during the past year, I wonder if it is the result of an event or action she could have avoided or bothered to.

Mary dislikes even the idea of sedation for pain. She says, "I have to keep active or I'll go crazy."

If someone senses that they are hanging on by their fingertips, why would they want to relax or let go?

It is unlikely that Mary's lifelong tendency to work vigorously and constantly will diminish just because I suggest it. She knows she needs to move with more care and has said as much. As yet, her behavior doesn't match that knowledge.

Mary's physical manner and speech are a perfect match. Her remarks are terse, precise, clipped, and carefully planned. She's not exactly joyful.

But, being human, Mary also possesses the ability to uniquely express herself in another way. Perhaps her garden displays this. What I need from her in therapy is some bodily expression that reduces her internal tautness and shifts her physiology from sympathetic dominance. In my experience this cannot be planned, and will not look anything like the swinging of a hammer.

My main job with Mary will be to help her understand that her tendency to work so hard is not the problem entirely. That behavior has kept her strong enough to prepare the ground for her garden. But for her pain, Mary doesn't need strengthening exercise and she doesn't need the immobilization that relaxing often implics. She needs corrective movement, and that must come from a part of her that she doesn't ordinarily trust and certainly wouldn't express in public. This part of her is spontaneous, graceful, and patient. Perhaps the best kind of therapy matches the patient's behavior and then shapes it without trying to eliminate it.

If I don't suppress Mary's natural enthusiasm for movement with criticism and disapproval, maybe corrective movement will blossom like those lilies she worked so hard for yesterday.

THE MAGICIAN'S MOVES

When you do cranial work, patients often use the word magic when describing their treatment to others. At first this offended me because I felt that my knowledge and technical skills were not being given the credit they deserved. Now I realize that no one was accusing me of anything, they were just commenting. (I remain sensitive about the term "voodoo," however.)

Nobody ever called me a magician when I was manipulating joints or exhorting people to strengthen their muscles. But I think just about everything happens for a reason or at least means something and maybe what my patients say these days can help me understand more about the nature of my work.

The essay "The Orphan" mentions archetypal psychology and I want to return to that theme here to explain a fundamental difference between a common method of management for pain and what I do today.

The archetypes or characters within us are often referred to as instinctive energies that emerge in behavior or speech. Any effort to keep them quiet results in their immature expression at exactly the wrong time.

The "warrior" is currently very popular in our profession. We buy machines that challenge our patients to pump up in ways unknown 10 years ago and the research journals are full of reports of the effects of strengthening on a variety of conditions. To some extent sports medicine is a fabrication of the warrior archetype, and a very valuable one at that.

But if I were in pain would I seek out a warrior to help me? Pain relief is not the warrior's job and expressing myself as a warrior wouldn't predictably ease my discomfort. Sure, I'd grow stronger, but I don't hurt because I'm weak.

The Greek god that is the equivalent of the "magician" archetype is Hermes. He carries in his hand the caduceus, the emblem of medical practice. Until a few years ago the caduceus was at the center of the APTA logo, but has disappeared. This happened at about the same time that the treatment for pain became mainly a combination of electrical stimulation and vigorous exercise. I'm not sure all of this is connected, but I remember how little in the way of magic my own practice had back then.

Think of a magician on the stage. He moves with grace, with power from his center, using gestures that have a special meaning and a quality of mystery. The spontaneous movement from patients that my handling reveals today looks very much like that.

On one level this motion can be understood to be simply that which is necessary to decrease the mechanical deformation responsible for the pain. I believe it is. But in another way it seems to represent a return to the archetypal magician, something rarely encouraged in a warrior's clinic. Are tai chi and Feldenkrais exercises the magician's moves?

One more thing—the major attribute of the magic is the ability to see patterns not seen by others. When movement in every direction seems to worsen the patient, but movement is the only possible way that they can resolve their problem, some corrective pattern must be found. Only a magician can see what to do.

It is as if the patient is lost in a thick forest and only the magician can see the path out. The following essay "In the Forest" addresses this in another way.

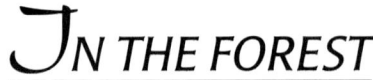IN THE FOREST

"The body assembles functions to point beyond itself."

Andrea Cartwright, yoga instructor/somatic educator

"I must have slept wrong or something, because my neck..."

Sound familiar? For anyone out there just beginning practice, you should be warned that this phrase will reverberate throughout your career. Even if you stop actually seeing patients, you will hear it anyway from friends or strangers who find out you went to PT school.

The insidious onset of stiffness in the spine might reasonably be considered the expression of a process and I have written of this many times. Lately though, something else has come to mind, something in the form of an analogy that my patients like more than my usual lectures on physiologic dysfunction. (I wonder why?) Here it is:

Suppose you were lost in a forest. The trees are randomly scattered and you wander for a long time without making any progress. Suddenly the forest begins to thicken. As your options for movement diminish, something becomes apparent—a path. In this situation it would be a welcomed sight. It should be remembered, however, that without a lot of trees, the path would never have been defined.

If you search through as many schools of bodywork as I have, you sometimes wonder how so many ideas about dysfunction and treatment could come from just one species. One common thread that runs through a lot of good work is that therapeutic movement or change has an effortless quality. Feldenkrais insists on this, Alexander wrote volumes about it, and yogic tradition depends upon it for every bit of lasting progress.

When the trees in the forest are scattered and few, I am not often aware of whether or not I'm trudging through the underbrush or cruising along the path out. If I start hitting tree trunks, unless I move with precision, it becomes easy to tell the difference.

Is it possible that we misinterpret stiffness as the problem when it really represents the solution? Might the brain organize our muscular function in such a pattern as to make any movement that was not corrective difficult? Surely we are smart enough to do this, and we will probably do it at night when we are less likely to consciously interfere with the thickening of the forest. Maybe dreams that help us understand our emotional life show up then for the same reason.

Many people live with chronic, low-grade restrictions to movement that never quite resolve and occasionally grow to include frank dysfunction and pain. In this state they occasionally walk into a tree, but most of their time is spent slightly off the path. The effort necessary to do this is mistaken for weakness, so they start lifting weights to relieve their pain (it doesn't help).

If a traditionally trained therapist encounters the patient in the forest, they might suggest modalities and mobilization. To me, this is like arming them with a heating pad and a baseball bat. Somebody else might tell them to lie quietly, hoping that the forest will disappear in time. Others offer something akin to chemical defoliants or maybe a chain saw. I think you get the point.

Let me be clear. I am suggesting that the unconscious mind creates stiffness specifically to make effortless correction easier to accomplish; easier because it is the only motion left us. This happens at least as often as I hear that comment about having "slept wrong." In other words, a lot.

We are all of us in the forest and it is time we looked at the trees in another way.

WHAT DO YOU THINK YOU'RE DOING?

"I just can't do it anymore. I've got constant pain in my wrist and forearm. I've started to drop things and now I'm feeling it in my shoulder."

The speaker is not a patient in my office, but a therapist at a workshop. In her face is reflected both the discomfort she experiences daily and the deadly knowledge that her favorite therapeutic tool has betrayed her. Her hands these days curl in, no longer reaching to treat patients, but unable to fully rest either.

Her history includes long periods of work on patients with heavy pressure. Specifically, this pressure was directed through a fingertip, a knuckle, or the volar eminences. It differed from joint mobilization where the hard elements of the patient are grasped and leverage is applied. She has just pushed hard and slowly, often gathering the skin in rolls as if it were as compliant as dough.

I seriously doubt there is a physical therapist anywhere who hasn't spent some part of his or her career trying to change one's patients this way. As a technique, it is common among a variety of bodywork disciplines and each has its own explanation for its use. It is commonly thought that heavy pressure mechanically distorts the myofascial unit in a beneficial way, that it promotes blood flow and relaxation.

But I've read of how transient this relaxation is, and whether or not the force applied actually travels to the target tissues in the direction intended is called into question in a recent article by Threlkeld: "If 100% of an externally applied force could be transmitted to the long axis of a connective tissue structure, manual therapy could produce permanent elongation...however, [these forces] are not direct and are not completely transmitted."

The ability of our bodies to disperse force makes it possible for an Indian fakir to lie on a bed of nails without being impaled. Of course, it is the vast distribution of weight along with the stillness of this direct pressure that makes it safe. Even a razor blade pressed directly on the skin will not break through without significant pressure. Movement enhances the razor's effect by overcoming the skin's ability to disperse force; the faster the movement, the easier the skin is to overcome.

I can't turn my hand into anything remotely as sharp as a razor. I can't make it sharp at all. My fingertips and knuckles are hard, but blunt.

With heavy pressure through them on a patient they become less like a hand and more like a weapon. By fashioning tools with our hands, humans moved from caves to condos. This had nothing to do with strength, but with dexterity.

If you look at the body's ability to distribute slow, steady pressure from a blunt object, you wouldn't expect "soft tissue work" to significantly alter any patient in a mechanical or structural manner. Still, we press on, usually in hopes that it will "work" by stretching or deforming something beneath the skin beyond its elastic range.

But often the changes that take place are most likely to be reflexive or circulatory, and there are easier ways to obtain these.

The damaged hands of the therapist at the workshop are not unique in my experience. They were wonderful tools used the wrong way. When I took shop in ninth grade and one day used a screwdriver as if it were a chisel, Mr. Ceresi grabbed my wrist, looked me in the eye, and said, "What do you think you're doing?"

Selected Reading

Morelli M, Seaboune D, Sullivan S. Changes in H-reflex amplitude during massage of triceps surae in healthy subjects. *JOSPT.* 1990;12(2).

Threlkeld AJ. The effect of manual therapy on connective tissue. *APTA Journal.* 1992;72(12).

THERE'S A DOOR

My automatic garage door opener malfunctioned recently. I felt a certain responsibility as a homeowner, husband, father, and supposedly competent adult male to see if I couldn't fix it.

I try not to rush into such things, because it's clear to me that my house anticipates my attempts to change it and then conspires against me. This is usually through subtle swellings or loosenings that resist the fit or attachment of any foreign object I buy at the store. My house has a remarkable immunity to such grafts, and now it seemed to be keeping me out as well. Pretty clever to use the garage door, I must say. I almost never walk home.

Years ago I had the image of my patients' problems being on the other side of a door. In order to affect them, I had to somehow deal with the door. In school I was taught to send waves of thermal energy, sonic waves, or electrical energy through the door. Early in practice, I learned how to use my hands to deform the door, hoping that the structures I needed to reach were close enough to the other side to appreciate my efforts.

Entering the garage from the house, I didn't get my stepladder out right away, but I did peer up at the mechanism for awhile. I know that there are wires and some kind of cable up there, perhaps just waiting for me to stumble within reach.

I found that my patients, especially those with spinal pain, had trouble that seemed some distance from any door I might choose. Their bodies had many entrances, but the structures I needed to change were smack in the middle. After a few years of pushing harder and harder, I concluded that that wasn't helping either. I'm a big, strong guy, but my own hands couldn't take it.

Yesterday I drove into my driveway and got out to lift the garage door. As I approached I heard the mechanism grinding away, trying to lift the door though I had released the cable that morning. Something had triggered the machinery without my pressing any buttons. It was mocking me. (And people try to tell me my house is not conscious of my presence.)

In the early 1980s, I watched several demonstrations of cranial work and submitted to a brief treatment. Something clicked. Something came together for me that included many of the theories and techniques I had learned and taught the previous decade. I could see that whenever I was effective with manipulation, muscle energy, counterstrain, functional technique, trigger point therapy, exercise, or massage, I had somehow passed through the door without effort. Somehow my technique became a kind of password that allowed me to enter the nervous system and elicit a reflexive effect that was far more powerful and therapeutic than anything I might do mechanically. For me, cranial technique became a discovery and refinement of passwords I might use on any patient. This is not just a matter of placement and pressure, but attitude and manner as well. My respect for the patient's ability to change is essential for success. When I was pounding on the door, I didn't feel this way.

As I stood in my snowy driveway listening to that mechanism grind away, it occurred to me that perhaps the opener in my car was at fault. Maybe it was stuck in the on position and had been continuously shouting at the door to open. This eventually creates some resistance in the wiring. Sounds like some of my therapy in the past. I changed the battery in my control recently and probably screwed the lid on too tightly. Nothing new.

The house is lucky I figured this out. I was about to go get my hammer.

$\mathcal{I}$T'S NOT ALL ARTHRITIS

I stood for a few minutes in a school parking lot recently and then sat in the auditorium for an hour. In this span I saw human motion near either end of its vast spectrum and I'm still wondering about it.

The occasion was my daughter Jennie's annual dance recital. I stood outside waiting for my aunt to arrive. Those of you with children in dance know that these events are attended by grandparents, great aunts and uncles, great-grandparents, assorted elderly neighbors, and the vaguely related people who transport them. Oh yes, middle-aged, anxious parents are there, too.

I watched a large proportion of the audience struggle from their cars, some of them lumbering across the gravel, breathing heavily on this hot summer evening.

Then, within minutes, I watched one class after another of young girls proceed onto the stage, displaying their skills in the disciplines of dance and the varieties of movement emphasizing jazz, tap, and ballet. Although the skill level varied, and many of the younger ones seemed to be dancing to tunes only they could hear, they all had one thing in common: they wanted to dance, and they did so proudly and without apology.

I know that aging inevitably reduces our range of movement, our strength, our quickness. I feel my own body going down like a ship when I measure it internally in these ways. But my attitude toward any movement is not a function of my age.

As an avid juggler, I will occasionally give lessons at local festivals and I always offer these at my workshops. At the festivals the children run forward, anxious to try. The adults hold back, using their age and "lack of coordination" as an excuse not to try. I know better. I know the adults are fearful of looking incompetent, foolish, or out of control. The psychologists call it "anticipated interpersonal disapproval" and I have felt it myself many times. My experience has been that juggling competence coincides with diminished fear of failure. Failure itself doesn't diminish, but the advanced juggler proceeds with increasing courage and isn't upset with all the drops.

I've found in juggling that people who are willing to keep picking up their drops eventually display the unself-conscious pride, poise, and graceful movement that the young girls displayed on stage. It is a fountain of youth for our attitudes toward movement, if not for our ever-aging bodies.

I watched my Aunt Alice coming toward me across the parking lot that night of the recital. She is not young, she is not light, but her step is. She almost floats, holding her head up, her eyes and face open and accepting. She has known the depths of life, but I know that these days she is content and happy as never before, and her movement shows it. She tells me that there is some arthritis in her knee, but I'm not concerned. She does not fear appearing less than perfect and this is displayed in her every movement.

Do we sometimes move poorly because we made a decision to stop dancing? Perhaps the posing of the adolescent is the beginning of that process that robs us of the spontaneity, courage, and poise of the young dancers on the stage.

The implications for therapy are pretty clear. We can't always reverse the consequences of aging on the inert tissues, but we can get the muscles to display a playful attitude. We should begin with ourselves.

By the way, the most beautiful dancer that night was named Jennie. And I wanted to be sure to mention that.

<u>Suggested Reading</u>
Dorko BL. Juggling courageously. *Jugglers World*. 1992;Spring.

THE SECOND LEVEL

"You know, someone said that the world's a stage, in it you must play a part."

Elvis Presley, "Are You Lonesome Tonight"

Michael Meade suggests that there are three levels of human interaction. The first level contains the simple greetings, common decency, and working agreements of polite society. It is dedicated to simple harmony and maintaining the status quo. Its bumper sticker is "Have a nice day."

The third level is the area of deeply shared humanity, fundamental oneness, justice, and transcendent functioning. A third level bumper sticker says "Visualize World Peace."

You may have guessed that the second level of human interaction is not as nice as those on either side. It is the territory of anger, conflict, vulgarity, sadness, and disappointment. I think you can come up with its bumper sticker on your own.

The reason I mention all of this is because I have for a long time wondered about the question, "How are you?" Despite my best efforts to the contrary, I am forced to ask this question several times a day and too often the answer makes me cringe.

Sometimes I get the first level answer, "Fine", when I am looking for something beyond that. Sometimes "Fine" is really all I wanted and I am hit with a list of symptoms and expressions of frustration that I am not prepared to receive.

Asking people how they are is a risky business. In the classic novel *The Trial* by Franz Kafka, the protagonist Joseph K. is in the midst of a terribly confusing and upsetting set of circumstances and accusations that have totally disrupted his normally mundane routine. A stranger on the street innocently inquires of him, "How are you?" and he is thrown into a prolonged fit of recrimination, renewed fear, and consternation. It is the result of a clash between the first and second levels of interaction, and I know I've done the same thing to patients in my office.

It is possible, at least to some degree, to maintain interaction on the first level by in some way making it clear that you don't want to hear any bad news. Do you know any therapists or physicians who manage this? I have long felt that without knowing it, therapists create a "play" in the clinical setting and choose their part and the parts their staff will play long before the patient arrives. The part remaining for the patient becomes clear sometime during the course of their first few interactions and for the most part they settle into their role. None of this is obvious and that is why it is so powerful. It explains why some therapists get three phone calls each day from patients wanting advice and I get as many in a year.

I think I tend to be a second level kind of communicator. Pleasantries are absolutely necessary to order society, but I want to move on. I know that unless discomfort is spoken of authentically, it will simply hide in the shadows until the worst possible moment. Perhaps the patient will wait and tell the doctor how awful they really feel and how little help therapy has been. Who needs that?

The second level may not be an easy path, but it can't be denied that it leads to the third level where acceptance, transcendence, under-standing, and human empathy may be found. There is no other path.

Elvis had a point. What's the play like in your clinic?

Selected Reading
Kafka F. *The Trial*. New York, NY: Alfred Knopf; 1960.
Meade M. *The Rag and Bone Shop of the Heart*. New York, NY: Harper Collins; 1992.

Suggested Reading
Dorko BL. *Getting arrested.*

THE IMPORTANCE OF CHOICE

In physical therapy there are many ways of approaching problems that appear to have much in common. This may be something that contributes to the confusion exhibited by the inexperienced clinician as long as he or she feels that among all the options available, there is only one ideal way of proceeding.

The fact is that many positive things can be said about most traditional and supposedly outmoded approaches to clinical practice, not the least of which is that empirical data supplied by the patient encourage the therapist to stay with it. In retrospect, it seems obvious that the human animal has an amazing ability to find a way of getting better no matter what the therapist did or thought he or she was doing. The common denominators among the many forms of care in therapy are just two: a patient in trouble and the presence of a therapist.

Choosing the approach to take to any problem may appear more difficult as our options increase. I have actually had students express anxiety when I point out some other way of treating their patients. They anticipate future conflicts with their co-workers, their patients who are used to the usual routine, and, most of all, within themselves.

This is understandable in a profession commonly urged not only to produce good results but also to move patients through the system with increasing speed and efficiency. Who needs a more thoughtful and reflective approach that will just gum up the works?

But there is another way of reacting to an increase in treatment options. Feldenkrais states, "Anxiety appears when deep in ourselves we know that we have no other choice—no other alternative way of acting." He suggests that we imagine how different we feel when walking along a 6-inch board lying on the floor and that same board suspended 10 feet in the air.

I have watched myself go through a cycle of clinical practice I feel is common. From school I began with a small number of approaches to offer those in my care. It was awful. As I learned more and expanded my options I felt better. I found one particular approach that seemed especially useful and I used it all the time. I felt awful again. I found and tried other options and felt better again. I figure I've been through this cycle about 20 times. I doubt that my patients have been essentially different in any way throughout.

I read recently of a top-flight rock climber named Lynn Hill. Aside from developing the physical skills necessary, this woman must continually confront the fear of falling. She does so by plotting her moves with precision and by exercising what options are available. As her choices diminish, the difficulty of the climb increases. It is interesting to note that rock climbers do not equate success with reaching the top, but with the climb itself. There is certainly the feeling of a hard climb in clinical practice. We will never reach the top. It would be wise to increase the number of options available.

Selected Reading

Feldenkrais M. *The Elusive Obvious.* Cupertino, Calif: Meta Publications; 1981.

New York Times Magazine. 1989;Dec 31.

MAYBE NEXT TIME

Gary lay on his back in the treatment booth in obvious discomfort.

"You know," he said, "this may sound crazy, but I knew that this was coming."

"How so?"

"My neck has been stiff and I just could not get it to relax."

Gary's pain and numbness were confined to low back and legs, as they had always been. After four lumbar surgeries, including the implantation of rods, he might expect some chronic discomfort. Still, I had not seen him for 6 months and he had felt perfectly fine. Three nights earlier he had bent forward to tie his shoes and the pain began.

Despite his surgical history, Gary works as a teacher, wrestling coach, and athletic director at a large high school. His schedule extends well beyond my own. At 43 years, he is 6 feet, 2 inches tall and weighs 260 pounds. Gary does not "tough it out" with any regularity; he does not ordinarily have any symptoms. When he begins to have pain, he comes to see me. Five or six sessions a year keeps him working and pain free.

The biomechanical reasons for a man of this size and with this history to have pain are obvious. If we only looked at Gary's chart and x-rays, we would expect him to be laid up much of the time and would never imagine that he worked vigorously at a full-time job.

But, Gary is graceful in his movement, quick to smile, and calm even in the maelstrom of a high school wrestling tournament. The famous philosophical dictum, "The map is not the territory," could be paraphrased here: "Gary is not his chart."

I have always treated Gary as if he knew what to do in order to get better. I do not poke at his back. I do not tell him what to avoid. I do not give him any long list of exercises. By now he has a clear sense of what his spine can tolerate and he does not want for activity or recreation.

The latest onset of pain reveals much about the nature of his condition, and his comment about his neck tells me that some of what I have told him in the past has begun to sink in.

I tell all of my patients that when they feel their muscles begin to contract, they might consider this not as an indication of trouble, but as the advent of correction. If they attempt to ablate this contraction with stretching or pressure or means of sedation, they usually end up with muscles in a prolonged isometric state. The consequences of this are well known.

What would happen if the patient trusted his or her system enough to let the unconsciously motivated contraction of his or her muscles become isotonic?

This is the way I treat Gary. In a variety of positions I indicate both manually and verbally that I trust what he wants to do. The end result is always the same. He returns painlessly to his life outside of my office.

Maybe next time when Gary's neck begins to restrict certain movements (what he calls stiffness) he will let it go where it wants to for a while. Maybe next time Gary will trust himself as much as I do, and later, when he asks for length in the spine, it will comply.

Maybe next time I see Gary, he will be coaching others and no longer looking for me to coach him.

ON TECHNIQUE

You may have noticed that I don't write a great deal about technique. It's not as if I don't know much about the subject, but rather that I feel very uneasy suggesting in this space that I know what another therapist's patient may need. I feel connected to other therapists enough to suggest ways they might interpret what they see and hear, but telling them where to place their hands, which direction to pull, and what to expect seems way beyond reason to me.

In a workshop setting I will certainly demonstrate technique. In fact, I spend a great deal of time speaking about the subtle but significant differences between one contact and another. But I find this not just difficult to do in a written form, for me it is an empty experience.

The director of academic affairs for the Rolf Institute is a friend of mine. His name is Jeffrey Maitland. In a recent interview Jeff makes a distinction between what we know and what we do. He says, "If I want to teach you checkers, I'd have to give you the constitutive rules or principles of the game. [These] tell you what moves are permissible and what aren't. If you violate any of these rules, then you're no longer playing checkers. There are also strategies that tell you which way to move under certain circumstances. You can ignore these, which means you're either very creative or ignorant."

As I read this, some of my problems with writing about technique became clearer. As my practice has evolved, my knowledge of the constitutive rules of human functioning has certainly grown, but there has simultaneously been an increase in my respect for the human quality of individuality and the changing nature of our being from moment to moment.

Let me give you an example. I used to think that the inert tissue of the body could be appropriately, adequately, and rapidly stretched if I just pushed hard enough or fast enough or long enough on the skin. I realized after a few thousand clinical trials, however (sometimes I'm a little slow on the uptake), that the body usually reacted to my pressure in the same way that those mushy balls in the novelty shops do, the ones that return to their original shape no matter what you do. My constitutive rules about the qualities of inert tissue were wrong and therefore my strategy was ineffective.

Actually, accepting the fact that pushing harder wasn't going to work was a relief. After all, I wasn't getting any stronger.

As I began to appreciate the significance of small nuances in my technique, I realized why descriptions or even pictures of technique would so often leave me cold. Meaningful demonstrations of technique for me included not what was said, but understood, not how the patient is grasped, but how he or she is released. These things are demonstratable but very difficult to write about.

My strategies these days arise from a newer set of constitutive rules about human functioning. Although these rules tend to shift as I gain experience, I can at least differentiate them from my strategies, my techniques.

Don Johnson writes of this distinction: "An education based on principles aims at freedom. Learning technique requires imitation...and obedience to those considered experts. Principles unleash ingenuity [and create] a community of explorers [while] an emphasis on techniques creates a society of disciples and masters."

Our profession has had would-be masters and it has had courageous pioneers. Looking at how technique is emphasized will help us distinguish one from the other.

Selected Reading

Johnson DH. Principles versus techniques. *Somatics*. 1986;Autumn/Winter.

Philosopher turned somatic educator: an interview with Jeffrey Maitland. *Massage Therapy Journal*. 1992;Spring.

BEATIN' ON THE DRUM

I played the snare drum from the age of 9 until I graduated from high school. Late in my career I was told of lessons given by the tympanist for the Cleveland Orchestra. I heard that during the first hour's lesson the student got to hit the kettle drum exactly once.

Having hit drums countless times for a few years, my adolescent mind thought, "What a ripoff!" Still, I never forgot this description of a lesson I never took, and today I think I understand why.

William Garner Sutherland, DO, would admonish his colleagues to "land like a bird" when they palpated the surface of their patients. I imagine that any bird knows before it lands what kind of movement is available to the surface it is aiming at. Landing on a roof must differ markedly from a wind-blown branch. Watching birds light effortlessly on remarkably disparate surfaces makes you appreciate the coordination they must possess. I wonder sometimes if they can actually plan their descent.

I have seen it suggested that grasping anything can be likened to an act of faith. Imagine unknowingly coming to the top of a darkened stairway, reaching out for the next step and feeling the jolt of this misstep reverberate through you. It is a moment of panic, a betrayal of faith.

How we feel when we handle something and how that something responds to our handling has a great deal to do with what we think is there. Like it or not, our patients clearly sense our lack of knowledge, our trepidation, the absence of our faith, and, being animated, they respond in kind.

Suppose I thought my patients were static, just lumps of tissue awaiting examination. I think that they would work to act like that and I would never get to see the subtle, unconsciously motivated movement of someone striving continually toward correction and homeostasis. If I do not know of or respect this tendency in those I touch, it will be impossible to see.

These days I try to land on my patients like a bird. I imagine the patient as an ocean, chaotic, occasionally ordered and periodic, driven to a wide range of expressions by the weather that it both creates and endures. Perhaps I can become a boat, respectful of the power beneath my hands, but able to navigate using my knowledge of anatomy and physiology.

As I said, I never took that lesson from the tympanist. I feel, though, that he must have known the importance of understanding what it was you were about to hit, its history and potential. That is why he played for the Cleveland Orchestra and I finished my musical career as a member of the Westlake High School Marching Demons. These days I drum on something than can drum back.

It really is a lot more interesting.

Selected Reading
Harrington D. Body of faith. *The Humanistic Psychologist.* 1987;15.

SILENCE

I recently read *Coming to Our Senses* by Morris Berman, a remarkable book that connects our physical experience of being in the world to the history of Western Civilization. He writes of things like the emergence and disappearance of mirrors and how this relates to society's sense of self and the subsequent codes and laws that were followed in different eras. He writes of cycles of orthodoxy and heresy and relates this to our bodily experience of feeling and how this is reflected in art ranging from cave walls to Disney cartoons.

It is a wonderful book and I couldn't recommend it more highly.

There are a few lines on the first page that struck me as significant to therapists and it seems they won't leave my head except out through my hand, so this essay came to be.

Berman recalls family gatherings in his youth that were full of warmth and reassurance. There was, however, something else: a complete absence of silence. Not silence of the hostile variety, but the kind that might emphasize simply "being" together. There seemed to be an unwritten rule that such silences were to be avoided because they might prove uncomfortable.

If silence results in discomfort, Berman suggests that it is because it exposes a "basic fault" in our individual ways of being. He means fault as in the San Andreas fault, the Void within that each of us faces only when both external noise and thinking stops.

He also points out that in other cultures, silence such as this is a comfortable fact of life and known to be therapeutic.

Having read this, I began to think about the use of silence as a modality in my office and found that it seems to come in different forms. It is important to distinguish between silence full of thought and something else. Brooks states, "The essence of sensory awareness lies in distinguishing our actual experience from our thoughts and fantasies." If we identify ourselves with the latter, we place a veneer of introspection (thoughtfulness) over interoception (internal sensation). What is going on inside is only evident when we feel, not when we think.

There is a kind of thoughtless silence when we are alone and, I think, another kind when we are silently with others. The tradition of meeting silently as a group is well-known among Native Americans, Quakers, Hasids, and many others.

While there is little doubt that such meetings are healthy in their own way, being silent with our patients in physical therapy adds another dimension to this meeting: enhanced sensory awareness secondary to touch.

Brooks again: "[Coming] to another quietly and without overt manipulation is normally very moving to the person who is touched. And [if] the one who touches is really present in what he does, he is apt to feel the wonder of conscious contact with the involuntary, subtle movement of living tissue."

It has been my experience that handling as described above often decreases thinking in favor of feeling, not only in the patient but in the therapist as well.

Maybe my lack of success at times has to do with my tendency to talk so much. By talking I "a-Void" the emptiness in me and simultaneously keep my patients from finding their own answers.

Sometimes, though, I face my internal experience along with the patient. Silence is the key to these moments and at the right time, and with the right patient, it provides light to solutions within each of us.

<u>Selected Reading</u>
Berman M. *Coming to Our Senses*. New York, NY: Simon & Schuster; 1989.
Brooks C. *Sensory Awareness: The Rediscovery of Experiencing*. Santa Barbara, Calif: Ross-Erikson; 1974.

THE LIST

Sometimes I stop for breakfast at a small restaurant between my home and the office. I have found that I am just coordinated enough to eat and write at the same time.

The placemats here are full of ads by local merchants. Prominently positioned at the top center spot this month a massage therapist has placed a list of words, initials, and phrases that (I presume) he hopes will snare some business.

I've seen lists like this many times before and I think that this is an especially good one. It begins with a relatively specific problem (TMJ) and rapidly expands to larger and less well-defined complaints like "sports injuries" and "stress and tension." It finishes with a flourish—"many diseases and disorders."

I can't say just exactly what kinds of massage this practitioner might employ for all this, but I wouldn't suggest that they won't help in some way.

Anybody who thinks that it is primarily the technique of handling that helps another is probably pretty new to practice. I lost track of the number of techniques I have used for a single diagnosis of low back pain and I have concluded that most of what I perceive of any patient depends upon how I choose to treat them. William Barrett wrote, "Technique has no meaning apart from some informing vision."

Dorko's Law of Vision and Coercion

"The amount of relevant information given the therapist is inversely proportional to the willful manipulation of the patient during examination and treatment, usually."

Often I wish that weren't true or, at least, not usually true. But I never saw my expertise or effectiveness grow in proportion to the size of my evaluation form, or the number of tests of provocation I performed or asked the patient to do.

Oliver Sacks says it beautifully: "Our evaluations are ridiculously inadequate. They show us deficits, they do not show us powers...when we need to see a being conducting itself spontaneously in its own natural way."

Now back to the list. I have no doubt that it is possible for this massage therapist to help the wide variety of conditions indicated. But I doubt that the passive movement of tissue accounts for all the improvement evident. In fact, the more serious the condition, the less coercion is done. My guess is that "many diseases" elicit in the therapist a careful watchfulness, a hesitance to act, and an openness to information that would be hidden under the barrage of traditional testing. I know this happens in my office. The list of conditions helped with simple therapeutic presence is pretty long.

I'm not sure we could fit all of them on a placemat.

Selected Reading
Sacks O. *The Man Who Mistook His Wife for a Hat*. Magnolia, Mass: Peter Smith; 1992.

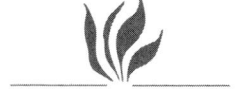

WHEN TOM SMILED

I was the last man on the eighth grade basketball team. This meant that I got into the end of games that were not exactly close. Okay, they were massacres, one way or the other.

If a player had a chance to shoot a foul shot, a cheerleader in our tiny gym would tumble and shout something in a singsong voice. I still remember from the single time I heard it directed at me.

"We wanna win, so put it in,
c'mon Barry sink it!"

My response was to throw up a total brick. Well, no big surprise.

At this same time I was in my fourth year of regular contact with a music conductor named Tom Hill. Tom would be the only band director I ever played for and in the band I didn't sit at the end of the bench—I was first chair.

A demanding, disciplined, and intense man, Tom loomed large in my life and was connected to the one thing I really excelled in. Like any good director, he would stop our playing whenever the sound didn't match his standards. This was quite often. I have never been interrupted so many times by anyone else in my life.

But at performance, as we sat self-consciously trembling before the first piece, Tom would step carefully onto the podium, turn to us, and smile. He smiled often, but this was different. I swear he saved this one for that moment. Its effect was to calm me and let me know it was going to go well, and I still feel it as I think of it today. Maybe my basketball coach did the same for his first stringers, I don't know. He never smiled at me.

Today I saw a man with two hearing aids and I had to shout a lot through the treatment. (I finally stopped shouting three patients later.) I always feel that I haven't done a very good job when this happens. To me, therapeutic presence for pain relief should not include a loud voice. When it's loud, my voice loses the subtle changes in expression that give the listener a chance to hear themselves. When I press hard with my hands, the same thing happens and the chance for the patient to feel it within themselves is lost.

Tom's "performance smile" is my model for behavior when I begin with patients in pain. At a recent workshop I demonstrated treatment on a student for awhile. When I stopped, a woman in the class said that I reminded her of a local orchestra conductor in the fashion I handled patients. She couldn't have given me a greater compliment.

I often state that the reflexive reaction to stimulus is more profound than the mechanical. Tom's smile never actually touched me, but its effect reaches across the years, as does the cheerleader's shout. Obviously, one was more therapeutic than the other.

I think I need to write Lenny Siwik and explain why I was such a pathetic player for him.

It was the cheerleader's fault.

WHAT DO YOU CALL THIS STUFF?

In 1910, a young physical educator in Berlin, Elsa Gindler, contracted tuberculosis. She was unable to pursue traditional care in a sanatorium and instead turned inward, attending carefully to her breathing and, eventually, every accessible aspect of her soma ("The body experienced from within," Thomas Hanna). After her recovery, she went on to develop many techniques of enhancing sensory awareness and thus produced what she called gelassenheit, meaning "allowing" in the physical body and "trust" in the psyche.

I talk a great deal to my patients about what may account for their problems and how physical therapy might help them and they often display a clear understanding of the care I provide. I can explain every aspect of a patient's sensory response to manual care via reflexive and mechanical processes well-researched and published in refereed literature.

In fact, I can bore anyone for hours with the intricacies of epithelial response to touch on a cellular level, energy transference in the neuronal tissue, and intratester reliability in palpatory diagnoses.

There is, however, one thing I struggle with: a name for what I do. When a patient in the midst of changing in response to simple contact says, "What do you call this stuff?", I am at a loss.

Now, unless you've been living in a cave for the past 5 years, you've heard of craniosacral therapy and myofascial technique. I have difficulty differentiating one from the other and even more trouble sorting out the subspecialties each of these methods offers at advanced courses. Maybe if I actually took a course one of these days, some of my confusion would lift. But I've listened carefully to many therapists thoroughly trained (and, in fact, now training others) in how to employ the techniques taught at these courses and I am struck by two things: a distinct lack of appreciation for physical law and a model of bodily functioning and expression that does not match anatomy or physiology as I know it. What I mean specifically by that has been addressed in many previously published essays and articles.

It is clear to me today that this work, although at times remarkably effective, has been tainted by outlandish claims of success and questionable theory. My essay "The Relativity of Wrong" addresses the problems inherent to this situation. I am often perceived as just another one of those spacy myofascial guys and it is a reputation very hard to shake. Saying I "do" myofascial release doesn't help.

Elsa Gindler established a very successful clinic and her work is now formally called "sensory awareness." Gindler herself refused to call it anything other than Arbeit am Menschen (work on the human being). Her discovery that kinesthetic awareness, however achieved, enhanced function, healing, and correction has been repeated countless times since.

When our work resembles this, it is simply the essence of physical therapy.

<u>Selected Reading</u>
Hanna T. What is somatics? *Somatics*. 1986;5(4).

Waiting

My mother tells a story of going to the doctor with my sister for her 1-year check-up. She was concerned, "Shouldn't she have some teeth coming in?" The doctor shrugged, looked at her, and said, "What are you gonna do?"

Mom was so struck by a simple fact that she remembers the scene 50 years later. The fact was, there was nothing that she could actually do, but waiting would work. (It did too. My sister still has all her teeth.)

In *Wild Mind: Living the Writer's Life*, Natalie Goldberg explains the difference between waiting and procrastinating; "Waiting is something full-bodied. [Having] worked on something for a while you are wise to step back. Waiting is when you are already in the work and you are feeding and being fed by it. Procrastination is pushing aside or putting off. It is thinking the moment is tomorrow...it is a cutting off [that] diminishes you."

In therapy, there are many opportunities to sense the power of waiting. Distinguishing the difference between waiting and wasting time requires some knowledge of how the body works, of what is happening beneath the surface that takes time and needs no overt coercion. If therapy is likened to a conversation, the therapist can be seen as a good active listener who doesn't interrupt another before the point is made.

Waiting is so powerful that we often lose patients to it. This happens when the physician says, "Lets not try therapy just yet. We'll wait a couple of weeks and see how you do with the medicine." Surely, there are times when the problem is resolved and the medicine is given credit. Therapists know that it was the waiting that did it.

If the patient is worse for the delay, we must assume that procrastination was chosen over waiting. Conservative care walks a tightrope between spending time by waiting and wasting time by thinking mistakenly that the time to act is tomorrow.

Productive waiting requires acceptance of the current situation as some movement toward correction or healing takes place in the time ideal for it. If you mistakenly assume something is broken and in need of healing, when in fact intervention to assist correction is really what should be done, something will be immobilized needlessly, perhaps even harmfully. Lending a therapeutic presence to the process of correction at the right time is something we all get better at with experience.

Problems with recovery might respond to the right answer to a simple question: "Should I be waiting for my patients, or are my patients waiting for me?"

Selected Reading
Goldberg N. *Wild Mind: Living the Writer's Life*. New York, NY: Bantam; 1990.

TEMPLE'S GIFT

My reading material often arrives in bunches and one subject is not obviously connected to another much less to my work in the clinic.

Connections appear in time though, and sometimes I feel as if they form the complex web of reasoning that drives my behavior as a therapist. As I read and work, some strands of the web weaken, others become stronger, some confuse me. I recently read two books that are unexpectedly, but unmistakably, intertwined.

Emergence: Labeled Autistic by Grandin and Scariano is the autobiography of Temple Grandin, a recovered autistic woman who has managed to both overcome and use her autism in order to become a highly educated and innovative animal behaviorist and inventor.

Temple describes the isolation, confusion, and fear that filled her childhood and adolescence. Her inability to process stimuli in a normal fashion led to the behavioral aberrations common in people with autism: uncontrollable anger, intolerance to change, obsession, and self-imposed withdrawal. However, Temple managed (with great difficulty) to progress through a number of private schools and at the time of her writing was completing work on her PhD.

I should mention that "recovered" in this case is a relative term. Temple's manner continues to set her apart and she maintains what she calls an "autistic logic" that makes normal sensory perception impossible. Her tendency to obsess over a device, an idea, or a symbol, however, led her to emerge from a particularly painful conflict within her world and offer something to ours.

From early childhood, Temple sensed a need to be embraced. Unfortunately, human touch, even a handshake, was intolerable. Like many stimuli, Temple says, "it went through my head like a freight train." She spent much of her life working to resolve this conflict and was one day struck by a sight at her aunt's cattle ranch.

As the calves entered the cattle chute they were anxious and hyper-reflexive, much like Temple. The moment they were held about the neck by a metal device they were calmer. Temple reasoned that a similar device would help her. This device would have one important exception, she would control the embracing herself.

She went on to develop a series of prototypes she referred to as "squeeze machines" that allowed her to rest inside a box and feel it compress her body while she controlled levers on a pneumatic device.

Temple found that regular use of the box not only calmed her, it somehow helped her for the first time in her life to experience empathy.

Although the beneficial effects of tactile stimulation are well-known to those in therapy, Temple's experience seems to imply that there is more here than we might have thought.

After I finished Temple's book I read Diane Ackerman's *A Natural History of the Senses*. The section on touch should be required reading for all caregivers.

To Ackerman the skin is the most remarkable and useful organ we own. It seems clear that when it is not stimulated in a nurturing way on a regular basis, we will pay dearly. This assertion is backed by numerous scholarly references. It is clear to Ackerman that therapeutic stimulation need not include another person; improved health commonly follows contact with inanimate objects as long as they are not perceived as threatening.

Temple's "squeeze box," which began by understanding the psychology of the cattle chute, is clearly validated in Ackerman's text. This autistic woman offers our profession a remarkable gift, an insight born of painful conflict and frustration, now ready for us to open and offer others.

Selected Reading

Ackerman D. *A Natural History of the Senses*. New York, NY: Vintage Books; 1991.

Grandin T, Scariano. *Emergence: Labeled Autistic*. Arena Press; 1986.

THE OLD GUARD

Paul, age 9, has had a terrible weekend. On Friday, he turned his head left in response to his mother's call and it stayed there. Acute pain, worsened with any attempt to move his head back to the center, has remained until now, Monday afternoon. He stands before me, eyes full of recent tears, nearly sleepless for 3 days, shoulders hunched, hands and arms curled up to his throat.

In Arlington, Virginia, "The Old Guard" marches before the Tomb of the Unknowns. Its members are remarkably the same in every respect. The precision of their movement is matched by the perfect stillness of their erect postures. Their presence lends dignity and a sense of ritual to any gathering. They seem to embody composure and stability. The public watches their performance silently, almost reverently.

Paul's mother is a nurse working for a local physician, so Paul was quickly and thoroughly examined before the doctor called asking for help. "He's stuck. Maybe you could do some manipulation?"

I, too, am drawn to any display of human precision and discipline, the kind The Old Guard offers. I like drum and bugle corps, drill teams, marching bands. There is something about a collection of humans moving and appearing as one that fascinates us so that we support them monetarily and emotionally. Most governments in this world have institutionalized such groups and use them as an exemplar of their tradition and power.

Paul's doctor is clearly concerned and I appreciate his confidence in my care. It has been suggested that Paul be corrected, that something be done to reduce this obvious deformity. In other words, the deformity is the problem and a return to the center is our first and foremost concern.

Paul doesn't care much about straightening out his neck. He just wants the pain to stop. He's been cold for 3 days and has asked repeatedly to lie in a warm tub. He is making absolutely no effort to return his neck to a neutral position.

As a fan of human precision and erectness, I feel an urge to coerce Paul back to a straightened position. I want very much to see him facing forward, composed and ready for movement, to make him look like a member of The Old Guard. I am in fact licensed to push him in that direction.

But many failures with coercive technique have taught me that Paul knows a lot more about what to do than I. If I accept his resistance to movement toward the center as appropriate, he will show me the path out of trouble. And if I listen carefully, he might just tell me how he got into such a fix. When I finally grow silent I hear of his roughhousing, go-carting, sinus surgery, a terrific fall from his bike. Paul has all the answers.

I have a friend formerly of The Old Guard. He tells me it's not unusual for members to wear girdles, use strapping tape to maintain their posture, or alter their boot heels to achieve a uniform height. Some of what the public perceives is an illusion. The uniform hides it well, and it is the only thing we can actually see.

Paul's posture wasn't much changed after the first visit; his shape was the same. But he was smiling, he was warm, and he felt real sleepy. If we suppress the urge to make him look better on the surface, his recovery will proceed in its ideal time.

When understood, the underlying, invisible processes beneath the surface are every bit as impressive as The Old Guard.

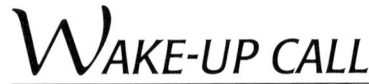

WAKE-UP CALL

"One does not become enlightened by imagining figures of light, but by making the darkness conscious."

Carl Jung

My mother worked for 17 years as a licensed practical nurse on the orthopedic floor of a small hospital. She once described to me the manner in which she wakened her patients early in the morning.

"I walk around quietly turning out the nightlights. They begin to stir soon afterward."

This is another one of those things that I heard long ago and somehow still remember. Fortunately, I have this space to explore the connection between these unforgotten descriptions and my work in the office.

Not long ago I was teaching at a pain clinic. As I watched the staff, it became clear that in this place the patients were welcomed, cared for, and listened to. It was a wonderful place.

However, as I watched, I became aware of something consistently done by everyone on the staff. While the patients spoke they were touched on the arm or the torso by the therapist and gently stroked or patted in a comforting manner. This seemed appropriate, although it's not the kind of thing I commonly do at all. I began to consider the messages that this kind of handling might give the patient. Things like, "I understand," "I feel for you," or "I'm so sorry you're unhappy." Then I began to consider some other possible messages, things like "Calm down," "Stop that,""I wish you were different," and "Be still."

At first glance these phrases don't seem all that bad. They imply caring and attention. Remember, nobody actually says these things, their fingers do the talking. In this way the message passes unspoken from the body of the therapist to the felt sense of the patient. These messages are everywhere so nobody has to speak them.

Do our patients always need treatments that tranquilize them or imply that their current activity is unacceptable and a clear example of what is "wrong" with them? Is manual care best used as a method of sedation or suppression of activity?

If we assume that people commonly go about living their lives in such a fashion as to make themselves worse, it makes sense to stop them, to change them with our manner, our grasp, our disapproving stroke or pat. We know that we can bend them to our will with nothing more than a subtle, well-timed look. Our touch says even more.

But if we imagine instead that the body is working toward homeostasis, we wouldn't ask it to stop what it was doing manually or otherwise. We would touch it in a fashion that asked for more of its essential, unconsciously motivated movement. Think of the body as a gift as yet unopened, and we want to save the paper.

Patting, rubbing, and stroking all have their place in manual care. But they don't waken the patient to the way he or she is at this moment, they encourage the patient to be something he or she is not.

We should watch that our manual care does not lead to the kind of things Sarge does to Beetle Bailey each morning. I'd like to think that our care might more closely resemble my mother's walk through the wards, making it darker so that people could wake up.

THE WIZARD

"Oz never did give nothing to the tin man that he didn't already have."

"I feel like I need oil." Clinton speaks to me while he moves about in an attempt to relieve his symptoms. Obviously, he doesn't know which way to go and the effort to escape his own system shows on his face, a face that is ordinarily impassive aside from this. The rigidity in his limbs and spine seems to reach past his eyes and I wonder what he's feeling aside from pain.

His remark about the oil reminds me of someone else asking for oil, someone I read about many years ago: L. Frank Baum's Tin Man in *The Wonderful Wizard of Oz*.

Although you wouldn't know if from the movie, the Tin Man's story is especially poignant and begins long before rain rusts him into immobility. He is an ambitious young woodcutter full of love for a Munchkin maiden (I'm not making this up). Working hard, he cuts off his own left leg with his axe. He gets this replaced with a tin one and then proceeds to hack off his remaining limbs, then his head and finally cuts himself in two, only to be successfully repaired each time by the tinsmith, otherwise known as the wonderful orthotist of Oz (okay, I made up that last part).

He admits that although his new parts take some getting used to, he is proud of his shiny exterior and the fact that he no longer can be hurt by the axe. The final repair to his torso did not include a heart, however, and he "lost all my love for the Munchkin girl."

I've seen my share of "tin men" over the years. Immobilized, injured at work, hardened by years of striving only to find that there is a certain emptiness left once their bodies betray them. Without their usual complement of movement, normal emotion seems diminished as well.

When Clinton came to me he had not been able to obtain a clear diagnosis or relief for his bilateral lower quarter numbness despite every available test. He even underwent a cervical fusion that helped none of his symptoms, although the surgeon assured him it would. I had helped him with Bell's palsy some years ago and he insisted that his family physician send him to me again. Whether or not I can help remains to be seen. I wish he could see a psychologist. No one will pay for that, and he is resistant anyway. This is what I have to work with.

In the book, the Tin Man admits to the Scarecrow that his brain is gone too, but "having tried them both, I should much rather have a heart." It's a great detail.

Now I get to play the part of the Wizard. In the book, the Wizard just places a heart made of silk and sawdust into the Tin Man's chest. I like the movie version better. You may recall that the Wizard insists that the Tin Man already has a heart and that all he lacks is a "testimonial." The Wizard says, "A heart is not judged by how much you love, but by how much you are loved by others."

Following this reasoning, I may have something to work with. I can show Clinton what he already has in the way of corrective processes. I can express my appreciation for his faith in my care. I can tell him that with what few powers I possess, I will try to make his journey to my office worthwhile, and that maybe once he gets "oiled," he can find his heart.

MOSHE'S AMBASSADOR

Previously, I wrote an essay about my partner's infant daughter, Alexis, coming to be with us in our small office. She was just a few weeks old and full of lessons in therapeutic presence and attention to the beautiful details of this world.

Now Lexi will tromp up the stairs to the room where I sit at my desk, shove open the door, and wait for me to drop my pen, pick up a harmonica, and play a tune. In response she dances about and claps at the end. It's like something out of an old Shirley Temple movie.

How different she is from anyone else around here, and how different I am in her presence.

More and more often, the physical therapy community is being made aware of the work of Moshe Feldenkrais. Perhaps hundreds of us have entered the training programs offered, attended lecture/demonstrations, or purchased the audio- and videotapes describing the movements he proposed would create new ways of functioning. But the essence of his message—that the brain naturally held the ability to change the way we placed ourselves in space and the key to unlocking new patterns lay in experiential, thoughtful, painless active movement—remains lost on the vast majority of therapists and virtually the entire medical community.

In 1981, I spent 4 days in the same room with 400 other people and one of them was Moshe Feldenkrais. He did all the talking. In the presence and under the direction of this man we explored our physical shadows, that is, the ways we usually weren't. He invited us to play, and we saw for ourselves how different we could be, and how unnecessary was pain and effort and goals and tests and documentation and judgment. It wasn't much like therapy as I knew it. And it will never be like therapy the way it is becoming.

Years later I wrote of Edelman's work on neuronal networks and how patterns of behavior influence our perceptions. I used this to explain why the physician could not see the patient as does the therapist and now I see in Lexi's behavior something more relevant to my clinical work.

What we describe as a functional brain, one that produces patterns of activity that get us through the day with relative safety and productivity, has gotten this way by stripping away the earlier patterns we had used to get what we wanted as children. Without schedules, deadlines, obligations, or a society to please, we might instead choose movements that please us, make us feel unique, competent, and whole. If these movements conflict with the expectations of others, they may be held within. All Feldenkrais suggested was that a therapist might provide the environment necessary to make such movements safe. He knew that they would help.

Still, there is little in the current literature on treatment that reinforces so radical a notion. We are offered protocols, regimens, more intricate testing, and then told to reduce our time with the patient in the interest of cost.

But in my office Lexi wants me to play another tune, and she wants to dance. Soon enough, she'll stop asking, and her movement will become more like mine, and maybe one day like a patient in pain.

When she comes to the door I pay close attention, and I hang on to her presence as I've tried to hang on to Moshe's.

Selected Reading
Dorko BL. Perceptual clarity in PT. *PT Bulletin.* 1989;Apr 12.

Suggested Reading
Dorko BL. *Alexis.*

SWING BAND

I spent some time near a waterfall in the courtyard of a Holiday Inn in Tampa, Florida, recently.

As one of the chaperons for my daughter's high school band, I had been assigned duty between 3:00 a.m. and 6:00 a.m. I think I was supposed to roam the grounds in search of adventurous teenagers but the only activity was that of the waterfall. In fact, I would have had to drag some poor exhausted kid out of bed in order to have any excitement. Clearly, Tampa was safe from the Cuyahoga Falls Tiger Marching Band. At least on my watch.

There are places in this world where there is at least the illusion of order, and that night the motel exterior was one. The perfectly symmetrical sameness of the architecture barely covers what I've seen inside those rooms, and the absence of sudden, explosive sound effects from many of the young men will not last 5 minutes beyond wake up.

Often this group is more like the waterfall a few yards away. Although it streams into a common pool, the movement to that point is loud and chaotic. But once ordered, this band can march and play as one, and they hear applause for that several times each day here.

In scientific terms, chaos is not random, wild, and unpredictable, but activity within a system that harbors an order in its overall behavior. We know that the human body has chaos lurking within its neural circuits, the beating of the heart and the flow of its blood. Health is the result of an ordered impulse that emerges from a variety of stimuli, each dependent on the others in numerous ways. It's as much an illusion of order as this motel at 4:00 a.m. or our band in a parade. It's nice, but it's transient.

The Tiger band is unique among the 18 assembled here. We are a swing band, and all the others are corps bands. A swing band flourishes their instruments, bobs their heads in the midst of full turns on the field, and lifts their knees when they march. Some drills require jumping in unison and looking toward the sky with the instrument held high.

Corps bands concentrate on small, tightly controlled steps, stillness in the upper body, and, it seems, an expressionless demeanor while in formation.

It seems to me that the similarity between this chaperoning and my clinical work is in the order and disorder I see melt one into the other several times a day. As a therapist, I try to organize my patients' movement into ways that will protect or strengthen them. Often I hear of their worsening when they moved "without thinking." As a chaperon, I herd this loose mass of teens from one venue to another, and then watch them move together with only the beat of the music needed to guide them. It's like watching the waterfall turn into a stream.

I'm convinced that I need to give my patients some freedom to personally express themselves as they march toward health. I know they have their own flourishes of movement that make them unique, and I prefer that.

I suspect that a swing band is easier to live with in the motel. They've left some exuberance on the field and the applause honors their individual movement as much as that of the whole.

Suggested Reading
Dorko BL. *The Old Guard.*
The mathematics of human life. *US News and World Report.* 1993;Jun 14.

THE SUPPRESSION OF FLIGHT

Instinct: a natural or innate impulse...natural intuitive power...urged or animated by some inner force.
Emotion: an affective state of consciousness.

Random House College Dictionary

Marie has come to my office holding her left cheek as if it were a small, wounded bird. It is Fall 1992 and I last saw her like this in early 1984.

"After you treated me I was fine until January 1991 when all my facial pain returned."

Marie went on to explain that 2 weeks before the return of her pain, her husband had committed suicide, employing a shotgun in the den of their home as she slept in another room. It was the dead of winter in Arkansas and an ice storm prevented her leaving the scene or help arriving for over 3 hours. "That" she says emphatically, "was stressful."

A remarkable article by Peter Levine details the instinctive physiologic reactions of prey animals to attack and inevitably capture. The well-known flight or fight response that ultimately mobilized the muscles for maximum power and speed is perfectly reversed once the animal realizes it is trapped. Prior to the killing blow of the predator, a mammal will grow limp, displaying a paralytic freezing evidenced by lower body temperature and profoundly diminished muscle tone. The trapped animal is not "feigning death" but rather reacting instinctively in a way that often inhibits predatory aggression. Animals do this naturally; humans must be taught that a bear in the wild may only sniff you if you lie perfectly still.

Marie suffered the pain in her face for 3 months. Then she heard through relatives of a surgeon who specialized in the management of trigeminal neuralgia and traveled a thousand miles for an examination. Sure enough, surgery revealed that her trigeminal nerve had been creased by a vein, apparently congenitally, and meticulous surgery restored her anatomy and Marie was without pain for 6 weeks. Then her pain returned.

Man's Presumptuous Brain by ATW Simeons, MD, traces the evolution of instinctive responses to threat and clearly differentiates these from human emotion:

"An instinct is a very old impulse which is generated in the diencephalon by a combination of hormonal and sensory stimuli. In this process the cortex is involved only to the extent that it censors the raw incoming messages from the senses. An emotion is the conscious or subconscious elaboration of a diencephalic instinct by the cortical processes of memory, association and reasoning. Emotions are thus generated in the cortex out of crude instinct."

Simeon goes on to describe the cortex as a censor of instinctive movement or expression. Beyond that, once the cortex transforms instinct into emotion it will commonly censor any expression of the emotion itself. He feels that since our society is built on cortical control as opposed to our basic instincts, psychosomatic illnesses will commonly occur. Only by identifying this conflict and accepting the complex working of our inner and outer lives might we avoid the insidious onset of chronic illness.

Marie's surgeon wanted to explore her nerve again. She was hesitant. "Maybe I just have a sinus problem. I'm going to the ENT clinic for another opinion." A massive infection was discovered; she was relieved of her pain with antibiotics and the surgeon dismissed her from his care.

Peter Levine has coined the term "fixated immobility reactions" to describe the array of clinical findings common among various, traumatic anxiety symptoms and syndromes. These findings are neuromuscular, autonomic, and perceptual, and predictably will accompany our instinctive response to intolerable or threatening situations. It appears that the entire scope of physiologic reactions to a simultaneous increase in parasympathetic and sympathetic tone became evident as Levine's technique of "somatic experiencing" enhances his client's awareness. Previously repressed sensations and bodily feelings are then used to transport the client through the event(s) as they are remembered in active imagination. During this process movement is encouraged. Levine states, "The central axis in the resolution of post traumatic and various anxiety responses was in completing previously thwarted motor acts...While catharsis (emotive response) may sometimes occur, it is the emergence of defensive activation that is the critical catalyst for therapeutic response."

After 3 months of pain relief with antibiotics, Marie underwent laser surgery for her sinus malformation. Her facial pain returned full force and the ENT clinic could not help her.

Simeons discusses the tendency for fearful flight as opposed to rage to predominate in humans. He points out that instinctive flight from threat is directly correlated to an animal's ability to bodily defend itself or counterattack. Humans have evolved in such a fashion as to nearly eliminate our ability to defend ourselves and the desire to flee with its attendant increase in sympathetic tone dominates the messages from our diencephalon. Cortical elaboration of these messages may result in a wide variety of emotions. These may be modified through cultural and sociological pathways so complex and embedded as to censure any overt expression of what we feel. We may suppress the feeling itself. The urge to flee lies buried beneath all of this.

It was suggested to Marie that she return once again to the dentist who had seen her in 1984. He adjusted her occlusion and she began to sleep normally and the pain receded. After 3 months the pain returned and the dentist sent her to me.

Levine has identified the need for movement to accompany effective care for anxiety reactions and the physical pain that is commonly concurrent. He refers to these movements as a "genetically endowed defensive capability." Appropriately expressed, these movements augment the emotion that may or may not accompany them. It has been Levine's experience (and mine) that a predominately emotive response to gentle handling tends not to be as productive as we would hope. It appears that care that reinforces dramatic expression of emotion rather than instinctive movement tends to recycle particular events without resolving the underlying conflict between the diencephalon and the cortex.

Marie is cold. She tells me she's been cold for many months. She realizes that her facial pain and her husband's death are no coincidence. Both of us know that during the 2-week interim between being trapped in a place she desperately wished to leave and the onset of her pain she did not change anatomically and treatment designed to alter her in that way has its limitations. It is time to move instinctively, and it's time to warm up.

I have nothing against the authentic expression of emotion. But I understand that by the time people are experiencing pain related to trauma and/or anxiety that the emotion they express during bodywork may be an elaboration of instinctive fear. What they need is movement that represents their effective defensive resources that were suppressed during the initiating event. Levine calls this "active-adaptive behavior." I call it spontaneous movement and find that it will emerge in response to "simple contact."

I ask Marie to move as she instinctively wishes, and she grows warm. Aside from an immediate decrease in her pain, she begins to sense a deep depression and drops the facade of characteristic cheerfulness she has maintained. She has work to do.

If I chose to do a body-based psychotherapy, I might seek more emotion and catharsis. But I choose somatics, a philosophy of care that emphasizes instinctive activity and the innate power of the human body to do the right thing with a minimum of cortical interference. When discomfort and dysfunction crosses that ill-defined border from acute to chronic, we need to look beyond joint mechanics and fascial restriction. If we take the time to examine the conflict each of us faces as both instinctive and emotive beings, we can begin to see more clearly what treatment should include. And we can keep the profession of physical therapy where it belongs.

Selected Reading
Hanna T. What is somatics? *Somatics*. 1986;5(4).
Levine P. The body as healer: a revisioning of trauma and anxiety. *Somatics*. 1990;8(1).
Simeons ATW. *Man's Presumptuous Brain*. New York, NY: Dutton; 1961.

Suggested Reading
Dorko BL. Persistent pain and underlying processes. *PT Forum*. 1988;7(25).
Dorko BL. The use of simple contact. *PT Forum*. 1988;7(16).
Dorko BL. The use of somatic philosophy in the practice of physical therapy. *PT Forum*. 1989;8(3).
Gellhorn E. *Autonomic-Somatic Integrations: Physiologic Basis and Clinical Implications*. Minneapolis, Minn: University of Minnesota Press; 1967.
Morris D. *Primate Ethology*. Wedenfield and Nicolson; 1967.

As TWO RIVERS MEET

There is a poem by William Stafford entitled "Turn Over Your Hand" that begins:

Those lines on your palm, they can be read for a hidden part of your life that only those links can say—nobody's voice can find so tiny a message as comes across your hand.

Manual care in physical therapy today has evolved into a complex variety of techniques and theories, often in marked opposition. For the many diagnoses for which it is said to be effective, the application of the hands to the skin ranges from heavy pressure with the knuckle to the gentlest possible touch with the finger pad. This is not an essay about what to do, but about what anyone touching others in hopes of being therapeutic might consider before he or she begins.

In his poem, Stafford takes an approach toward the palm of the hand that reveals his respect for its quality of shape. We know it to be unique and immediately accessible should we only take a moment to look. However, our habitual postures don't often expose the palm to our vision or the vision of others. In order to see it we need to consciously lift it open, as if opening the lid of a box. When we want to reveal ourselves to others we open our palms toward them, place our palms against theirs, or touch them in some fashion with the padded, more sensitive part of our hand's anterior aspect. On balance, it is the back of the hand that is used forcefully toward others, and that includes supposedly therapeutic techniques as well.

Stafford takes an approach to the lines of the palm that requires self-examination. He does not suggest that anyone else can tell you what these lines mean, but that they speak of a hidden part of our life that only we ourselves can sense. I would paraphrase the line to read: "Nobody else's voice can give you so true a message as comes across your own hand."

In short, this poem begins with an invitation to reveal a part of your life you normally hide with pronation and flexion. The act of supination and extension evokes feelings of vulnerability, openness, and supplication that many find too revealing to commonly express. Stafford's admonition, "turn over your hand," is both an unusual act and a movement toward revelation.

The skin is normally thought of as a barrier between the therapist and the organs they hope to affect with the various pressures of technique. In fact, however, it begins embryologically in the same layer as the nervous system and can be accurately described as the exposed nervous tissue, providing not a barrier but a bridge to the organ responsible for the sensation of comfort or pain. What the skin reveals in its temperature and response to provocation may be interpreted as a reflection of much more deeply embedded and widespread processes. A tender spot on the surface is often the tip of the iceberg, and not necessarily a reliable representation of a specific lesion or a good place to apply treatment.

The skin is our surface. Here we reveal what we may or may not want to, and here we often hide what we want most desperately to express. Similar to a river, its surface is fractally shaped, meaning that its intricate geometry is self-similar across scale like a variety of waves produced by turbulence, weather, span, rate of flow, and untold other influences.

Anything fractally shaped has been produced by chaotic forces and its response to provocation is simply not predictable. Although some fractals are far more stable or imbued with negative feedback than others (i.e., a rocky coastline), human skin is notoriously fickle in its ability to mediate underlying changes because of its connection to our mind. Consider the scope of reaction we may have when touched by the people we know (or don't know) in this world, even if the pressure and location of that touch were always identical.

When our skin is touched two reactions always occur: mechanical and reflexive. The former is a function of the amount of pressure brought to bear and it grows directly in proportion to that pressure.

Reflexive reaction is dependent upon the anatomical relations of the nervous tissue stimulated, and grows in inverse relation to the force of the pressure. It follows that gentle pressure is more likely to evoke widespread nervous reaction as well as a diminishing protective response.

Gentle touch reveals the body's "watery" nature and heavy pressure its rocky coastline.

Stafford continues:

Forbidden to complain, you have tried to be like somebody else, and only this fine record you examine sometimes like this can remember where you were going before that long silent evasion that your life became.

If the skin in its most intimate shape can be used as a metaphor for our true selves, and as an expression of that self through gesture toward and contact with others, it is also a reminder of the ways we aren't in the world. This is the "silent evasion" that Stafford suggests might be evident during thoughtful inspection of our own palms.

When we touch another we enter a place where we may or may not be welcomed, and this is not entirely dependent upon our approach or intent. Others have their own agenda, and may not find something in us with which they can resonate.

Bodily processes are often chaotic and this means that a tiny provocation can have a large effect, or, conversely, a strong provocation may produce very little lasting change. Predicting how anyone else will react when we touch them is, to put it mildly, a tricky business.

It would seem that gentle contact with the palmer aspect of a soft and pliant hand would most likely lead to an expression of self-hood that is authentic and therapeutic on several levels. There is no reason that the reaction mediated through the hand of the therapist shouldn't have a similar effect on the caregiver.

Perhaps those of us who choose to provide manual care should begin with the premise that we ourselves will be changed each time we treat another. It might make us think more carefully about our choice of technique.

In one sense, when we touch another, two rivers meet. We cannot manage them with force and coercion. We cannot account for every swirl and eddy, while at the same time we ignore them at our peril.

When we choose the simple modality of touch we influence directly an organ that both protects and reveals other organs, processes, thoughts, and feelings in ways both subtle and obvious, predictably and unpredictably. As William Stafford suggests poetically, the skin itself carries in its peculiar way the story of human possibility and the ways we might be if given permission. Perhaps the permission needed to move toward health can come from a caregiver who understands the potential power of simple touch.

Selected Reading

Cyriax J. *Textbook of Orthopaedic Medicine*. Vol 1. Baltimore, Md: Williams & Wilkins: 73.

"The least reliable way to diagnose in soft tissue lesions is to palpate immediately for tenderness in the area outlined by the patient." Increasingly, "trigger points" are understood to be transient physiologic processes and not visible anatomic lesions. Subsequently, techniques that seek to alter physiology through corrective movement, breathing, and expression are more likely to produce lasting results. Tender areas are at times useful as "doorways" into the sensorium by virtue of the membranous tension within the epithelium.

See "The Intimate Sense: Understanding the Mechanics of Touch" by Frederick Sachs in The Sciences, Jan/Feb 1988. Also, "Simple Contact and Distant Change" by Barrett L. Dorko. Unpublished copies available from the author.

Dorko BL. *Changing*.

Dorland's Medical Dictionary. 27th ed. Philadelphia, Pa: WB Saunders; 1988.

Arndt-Schulz Law: "Weak stimuli increase physiologic activity, and very strong stimuli inhibit or abolish activity." Also applicable here is Weber-Frechner's Law dictating that thresholds of sensitivity decrease in the presence of low excitation, thus enhancing interoception and the possibility of learning with gentle technique.

Goldberger A, Rigney D, West B. Chaos and fractals in human physiology. *Scientific American*. 1990;Feb.

The skin is specifically identified as fractal in "Chaos: To See a World in a Grain of Sand and Heaven in a Wild Flower" by Goldsmith. (*Archives of Dermatology*, September 1990.) See also "The Shapes Within" by Barrett L. Dorko.

Montagu A. *Touching The Human Significance of the Skin*. New York, NY: Harper; 1968.

Stafford W. *Stories That Could Be True*. 1977.

FOCUSING ON THE THERAPIST

To some degree, every job changes those who do it. If we choose our work of our own volition and find that it provides for us some significant measure of self-expression, then that change will include a way of being that includes what we desire.

Joseph Campbell remarked that if we can see a path clearly laid out before us, we should realize that it is not our path. Each step we take into our life's work might be given the energy of its force by some personal desire to move, but that doesn't mean that we know where it will take us, or that we would choose our experiences if we could foresee them.

In other words, the path a therapist takes will also include things we didn't plan on, and changes in our ways of being that we might not want.

This is unavoidable. I deal with it by writing about it and sometimes that turns into an essay. The following are pieces that relate to the changes I've been through as the end result of my career choice.

I don't know what may come with my next step along this path or whether I'll like it. But I am compelled to remain a therapist seeing patients, and I feel certain the life I'm living while in the clinic remains my own.

BRAD

Brad is my son's best friend. They are perfectly 10. By that I mean that their idea of entertainment ranges from "Terminator 2" to "Lambchop's Play-Along."

Last March, Brad suddenly became feverish and large blisters broke out covering his hands and feet and face. His throat was similarly affected and swallowing became impossible. He was hospitalized and a diagnosis of Stevens-Johnson syndrome was made. This is a relatively rare viral infection and defies most treatments aside from time and rest.

Brad lay in bed and suffered as you might expect while doctors and nurses trooped through, offering pain or sleeping medication. They took pictures for the medical journals and tried to learn about a disease most had not heard of before.

My career in therapy has not taken me close to sick children to any extent. I treat comparatively mundane orthopedic problems, pain with obvious origins, clear prognosis, and predictable consequences. Brad worsened, recovered slightly, worsened again, began tubefeeding, and was listless and seemingly beyond any more effort after 2 weeks of care.

At the Will of the Body by Arthur Frank details the author's observations of his treatment for and recovery from cancer. Frank's description of "caregivers" and "wonder" took me back to those evenings with Brad when my family would visit.

Frank defines caregiver as "[one who] is willing to listen to ill persons...and understands how each of us is unique. Care is inseparable from understanding, and like understanding, it must be symmetrical."

The symmetry that Frank refers to includes equal measures of third and first person awareness. Caregiving requires that when I listen to another that I hear myself, that when I see a young boy ill, I clearly imagine my own son in his place. I found this easy to do.

Treatment and care are not necessarily the same thing, although treatment is no less important. But by comparison, those who only treat choose to see the ordered sequence of illness experiences while caregivers are confronted with "the stew of fear, uncertainty, denial, disorientation, and bargaining" commonly felt and expressed by the seriously ill.

Since I had no treatment to offer (for a change) I could only care, and, predictably, it has improved me.

Frank speaks additionally of wonder. By this he means a shift in our perception of the body as a territory that the doctors or even our own consciousness controls to an entity beyond our control that we can only observe from some distance, and can only vaguely guess at its motivations or mechanisms. The body's own wisdom is sufficient and there is a time to relinquish our illusion of control and simply watch in awe. We cared and we watched and we waited.

I think that I knew Brad was really coming around when he and my son were again pretending together on the back porch. Initially sensitive about his appearance in front of other friends, Brad never hesitated to invite Alex into his room. He knew a caregiver when one showed up.

I'm coaching a local baseball team this summer and sometimes Brad runs up to me and asks to play shortstop or to pitch. "Sure," I say, "Go ahead."

Selected Reading
Frank A. *At the Will of the Body*. Boston, Mass: Houghton Mifflin; 1991.

ADDENDUM 1995

Brad was hospitalized during the NCAA basketball tournament and Ohio State was advancing. He and his mother watched a few games and, as those things will do, Brad found some relief in the excitement of a game he loves.

These days I watch Brad bring the ball up the court for his seventh grade basketball team. When he goes to a right handed dribble he always holds his left forearm across his chest as if protecting his heart.

He's a wonderful player, not tall or especially fast, he's one of those kids that can see the court, knows the game, and is a deadly shot.

He passes the ball to my son Alex, the other starting guard on the team, and together they run plays and sometimes struggle against taller or faster players. Whatever happens, they walk off the court together, and their fathers watch.

MAN TO MAN

Mike is short and rotund. Formerly a federal marshal and sheriff's deputy, he now has his own business making ammunition and explosives. His remarks about the government, politics, and hunting (he calls it "killing something") make it clear that we don't share much in the way of personal philosophy and I keep my mouth shut. This seems not to discourage his commenting on a variety of topics of his own choosing.

When I can sneak in some questions and examine him, it's clear that his recurrent spinal pain includes no pathology and should respond quickly to a little manual care and exercise. I'm not concerned about helping him with his pain, but I worry about getting through a few sessions without provoking him somehow.

I've spent a lot of time meeting with other men the past few years. I read all the contemporary literature about the recent movement of men together to reduce our isolation from one another. Along with three other men, I lead retreats that focus on the common problems and opportunities that being a man in modern times offers us. It's hard work. It's often painful. It's the best thing I do.

I've learned that the first thing the majority of men feel when in relation to other men is fear. If fear is considered an instinct rather than an emotion, it will be accompanied physiologically by sympathetic dominance and psychologically by a range of emotions, all of them negative.

Mike seems suspicious of my tendency to handle his limbs gently. He tells me of his numerous visits to the chiropractor and he's certainly used to and expectant of forceful manipulation although it never relieved his pain.

Mike's body is easy to change with treatment. He moves instinctively in a corrective fashion the moment I touch him, and does not object to my explanations or suggestions about things he might change. I have the feeling that I am getting more cooperation and change out of this man than most people do. (You should hear him speak of his fellow drivers on the way here.)

Mike was an adviser to the Vietnamese in 1963 ("some advice," he says), has been shot twice, and still carries a load of buckshot in his lumbar region. After a few altercations with prisoners, he left the sheriff's department in a hurry and seems to have a "survivalist" mentality that colors most of his statements about others and the future.

Mike likes me. I think he sees me as one of the few nonthreatening men he's ever met. I haven't mentioned his obesity and although he has yet to do any of the exercises I suggest, I accept the excuse that there is too much work to do. He says it's because of the Brady Bill and I believe him.

Our paths have been different to say the least. I've never been shot at or physically attacked. The closest I ever came to military service was the high school marching band.

Still, my manner has allowed both Mike and I to see how we're the same. I told him we both make money when others become fearful and he agreed. He told me that he loves Wagnerian opera and has a copy of the entire "Ring Cycle." We both think "Jeremiah Johnson" was a great movie.

A few years ago we would have clashed and I'm sure I would have felt that it was because Mike was a jerk and nothing else. Taking the time to be with other men and facing the fear it produces has shown me the common ground my gender struggles to find each day. It certainly makes it easier to help a man like Mike.

A COMMON GROUND

If you were to look at the pile of reading material I go through in a week, you'd wonder about some of its relevance to my work or my essays. My desk is strewn with items including volumes of poetry, harmonicas, half-finished articles for several publications, and a Mexican sun god from my twin sister in Philadelphia.

I've found that I can't go downstairs to the treatment booth without taking bits and pieces of this pile with me. Like every therapist personally managing patients manually, I express my unique knowledge and biases each time I touch somebody in an effort to change them for the better. Beyond the techniques of examination, I feel pressured to provide correction and relief with simple handling and this is often a daunting, if not impossible, task.

If I confine my attention to the tissues alone, I can carry on endlessly about the cellular nature of the nerves or the common misinterpretation of muscle function (this last one is my own idea).

But beneath the surface anatomy and beyond the reflection of nervous stimulation, I always discover a unique and biased individual with a cluttered desk (and mind) of their own. Where we meet, some accommodation must be made, and I can't help but notice things seemingly irrelevant to their complaint of pain or supposedly unrelated to their restricted movement.

Don Hanlon Johnson has written an amazing book about the influence of culture and personal history on the ways we move, feel, and appear. It is entitled *Body, Spirit and Democracy*.

In many ways, Johnson expresses a profound and personal appreciation for the human body that is born of the dramatic events in his own life and training as a priest, Rolfer, teacher, and philosopher. You could say that his life and extensive travel have been very different than mine, although my growing up in suburban Cleveland had its share of drama as well.

Still, he concludes that whatever he might bring to a therapeutic session is no more important than the inner life and workings of his patient. He knows that his vast store of experience cannot tell him what his patient needs to do in order to reduce the pain in their body, or find some peace when the pain is intractable. This must come from the patient themselves, and I agree wholeheartedly.

One statement he makes early in the book bears quoting: "Religious, philosophical, and therapeutic ideologies would have people believe that the way they stand in their peculiar space is a source of error to be corrected by reliance on officially sanctioned perspectives."

Often by remarkably different routes, those of us faced with the problems of human pain and dysfunction approach a common ground. Here the therapists and those in their care meet, dragging the clutter of their lives and their society with them. Don Johnson shows us how he lives in this place with its confusion and uncertainty, and how not to feel alone there.

Selected Reading
Johnson DH. *Body, Spirit and Democracy.* Berkeley, Calif: North Atlantic Books; 1994.

Suggested Reading
Dorko BL. *The ideal body.*
Dorko BL. *The view from inside.*

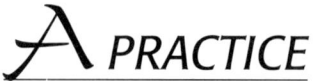 PRACTICE

Often when I teach, therapists ask me what exactly is it that I say to patients prior to and during treatment. "How do you set the stage?" was the way one woman recently put it.

I can't pretend that this question doesn't bother me. First of all, I can't really answer it because I'm sure I don't know. I have a variety of conversations with my patients. Who doesn't?

Evidently many therapists live in the hope that one day they'll be told exactly what to say and how to act so that each treatment will proceed in an orderly fashion. I say, "Good luck."

Sometimes I wonder why so many in my profession are anxious to be told what to do, what to say, or how to act. Commonly these therapists have been practicing for 10 years or more. They've seen thousands of patients. They have a wealth of clinical research readily available to them and they've attended more workshops than they'd like to admit. Still, they feel that there is in the behavior or words of some other therapist a formula for success that they haven't or won't discover on their own. They say, "I want someone with more education, more experience, more skill, or specially acquired knowledge looking over my shoulder to make sure I'm doing it right." I wonder if this is common among other health care professions. I suspect it is not.

Maybe this common desire to be told what to do is somehow connected to the large number of therapists I find at courses who suffer from as much chronic discomfort as their patients. Having found that their own methods of care are not helpful, they resign themselves to the pain and only seek relief fitfully, usually at weekend workshops.

Psychologist Sam Keen suggests that among our basic rules for living we include a persistent tendency to trust in our own ordinary experiences and to authorize our own life. It is, after all, the only one we must decipher. When we do this, we stop seeking authority and we become one instead. To do this competently, we must think hard, deliberate, and cultivate doubt.

I'm not suggesting that teachers can't help us understand the things we can't see or see familiar things in a new way. But how to impart that information to patients and how to behave must come from somewhere in the center of each individual therapist. Amid the complexities of the clinic we can only start with exactly what we have, and only our personal experience can help us.

In an essay I quote to all my classes, Heckler says, "A practice is not so much about achieving a goal, avoiding something, improving yourself, or making your wishes come true, but about creating a positive environment, internally and externally for the awakening process to take hold. A practice provides a path we may walk on, fall from, stand again, and relate in a direct and vivid way to others and the experience of our life. Choose a practice with a heart and wake up."

I would add that what we have to offer our patients is our unique presence. We can't get that from anybody else. It comes from what we see, remember, and believe. Don't ask anyone else for that. Find it in your own life.

Selected Reading
Heckler RS. A holy curiosity. *Somatics*. 1990-1991;Autumn/Winter.

DEVASTATION

"I don't think you really know what's wrong with me and I don't think you know what you are doing. What you've said and done here makes no sense."

I hear remarks to this effect about three times each year. That number is a guess, of course, but I'm confident of its accuracy. I say this because each time I hear this it has a profound and lasting effect. I feel shaken, stricken with uncertainty, angry, and self-righteous. That night, sleep is difficult and my thoughts continually turn to the patient, the symptoms, the referral source, and my methods and behavior. It is an experience both rare and profound. I notice it, and three times in a year sounds right to me.

If a therapist never hears these remarks, I would imagine it's because they aren't really seeing any patients. Either that or they have so insulated their clinical practice with layers of aids, assistants, modalities, and protocols, that the patient's opinion of their care is not possible for the therapist to hear. Sometimes the care is so regimented and generic that the patient has no idea to whom he or she might complain.

I teach a kind of handling that is fairly easy to learn and certainly seems effective and scientifically defensible. In class, people often change dramatically for the better, and they speak to me of how anxious they are to try this approach when they return to the clinic.

But I've spoken to many former students and found that, though the course was a pleasant experience, they never really applied the techniques as I demonstrated or suggested. They are vaguely apologetic and cite the conservative attitude of their co-workers, superiors, and the local medical community. They tell me that many patients object to gentle, thoughtful handling and insist that therapy be powerfully coercive or even painful. This last one I find hard to believe.

I think the tendency not to use gentle handling, though we know it may help, lies in the devastating effect the patient's rejection may have. My students say, "Okay Barrett, suppose I do this and the patient doesn't get better? Suppose they think I'm crazy?"

Although rare, I know that this can happen, and I can't pretend that such rejection is easy to stomach.

Manual care exposes us to such a situation far more commonly than simple, traditional regimes of heat and exercise. A practice that reduces the risk of rejection because the therapists never express themselves personally or uniquely through their manner or handling might be busy and successful in many ways, but it lacks something I want in my work.

When we handle another gently, we are on some level displaying an admiration for the ways that they are. When they move spontaneously and we accept that as appropriate and corrective, we draw even closer to their unique being and the walls that normally separate us become thinner. This opening simultaneously makes it easier for the therapist to see the problem and its solution while becoming more vulnerable to the patient's rejection. I can appreciate why most therapists would choose not to risk it.

This is not a solvable problem, and I only recently came to the conclusions in this essay. The impetus was another comment from a patient as I mentioned. For awhile, every compliment, every successful outcome pales in comparison. Writing this will help a bit, but I struggle to find the courage to open myself once again and start another day in the clinic.

JUMPING IN THE WELL

The varieties of care recommended for the single diagnosis of spinal pain have not decreased in the 20 years I've been in practice. In fact, I'm pretty sure most things we no longer do have been replaced by two or three new procedures. New essential diagnoses implying specific dysfunction in certain tissues create more procedures and these give rise to new regimes and protocols.

In turn, specialists, specialty clinics, and certification for competency through continuing education courses became necessary for conditions not known to exist a decade earlier. Well, sometimes the conditions weren't common, but that probably isn't true of backache.

Many therapists are critical of care offered elsewhere and I'm no exception. I have trouble with care pursued just because it "works" or when I find its theory illogical. I am not satisfied with traditional methods just because they fulfill the expectations of the physician or the patient. This has gotten me into trouble more than once, but I get around and I know I'm not alone.

But I have a very high regard for many therapists treating the same conditions that I see in ways I wouldn't dream of using. Notice I said that I admire the therapists, not the therapy.

Many of the therapists at workshops or conferences I attend take careful notes and watch me work with remarkable intensity. I know what they are hoping for, because I did much the same the first few years of my career. I was hoping that a certain lecture or technique would make things clear in the clinic. I was wishing that when I returned to handling patients they would respond as they did for Paris, Mennel, Kaltenborn, Grimsby, or Rocabado. I even taught courses with all of those men. I always wished my patients had been there.

But exposure to a variety of techniques taught me more about perception than skill. I came to understand that every patient, in fact every person, could display dysfunction in any way I chose to see it. One way or another, testing revealed my bias and treatment simply followed suit.

Ralph Strauch states in *The Reality Illusion*, "The people in your life are not your creations; they are separate beings, each as powerful and autonomous as you. [But] you create your experience of them, just as each of them creates his or her experience of you."

If this is true, and I believe it is, then my desire for clarity through testing would only rarely be fulfilled. Maybe this is why intertester reliability in manual care is so commonly poor.

The therapists I admire have not abandoned their efforts to know what is wrong, but they know whatever they think they see is just a small part of the total picture. They know the patient they don't help might have done well elsewhere, and even the ones they help might need more than they can offer.

After some period of experimentation, during which they discovered many ways therapy does not work, they came upon a method and philosophy that resonated with their unique experience of others. These therapists then deepened their understanding of how a certain theory leads to outcome, and how a technique accounts for relief.

Prior to that moment, each course attended was like a wishing well. They stood at the rim and looked in, throwing coins, hoping for all the answers. But sometimes a therapist is compelled to stop throwing coins and jumps in instead. Such a leap is followed by the courage to authorize our own experience, our own perceptions. When we choose this, we study and deepen what we do more each day. The profession can only benefit from such a leap.

Selected Reading
Strauch R. *The Reality Illusion*. Barrytown, NY: Station Hill; 1983.

Suggested Reading
Dorko BL. *Getting arrested.*

CHANGING

In an old episode of "M*A*S*H", a war correspondent asks questions of the hospital staff. In response to "Would you say you have been changed by this experience?", several cast members speak of the profound effect the circumstances and patients have had on them. When the camera lands on Frank Burns, he snorts, smiles, and says, "Certainly not!"

The literature regarding the effect of manual care on the patient grows remarkably each year and I can't keep up.

Some techniques even seem to transcend the patients themselves. That is, someone may be described by the method or theory employed to treat them. For example, I hear therapists at my courses say, "I have this McKenzie patient," or "She was a myofascial patient."

I have begun to wonder if such a description does not have some significant effect on our ability to see the unique qualities each patient might have. I wonder if a patient assigned to a certain method of care would be allowed to progress or change in any unexpected way.

We all know how some physicians or therapists who get it in their heads that a certain pathology or dysfunction would account for most of their patients' complaints. I have often done this. It makes practice easier for a while. This is soon followed by a mind-numbing boredom.

I think that our techniques of care or theories of dysfunction can, in some way, produce in patients the findings we want to see, and force them to progress in the way that we expect. It is a situation deeply rooted in human psychology and the power of projection.

Perhaps we can avoid this trap if we consider how the care of another might affect the caregiver. After all, I cannot touch another without being touched myself. Although this contact is confined to my hands, it could be argued that it is precisely there that it would have the greatest effect on my sensibilities. Being a manual therapist, my contact is likely to be prolonged and therefore more profound. When my touch is gentle, the reflexive reaction it may produce in the patient grows and need not know any boundaries except the furthest reaches of their nervous tissue. Heavy pressure diminishes the scope of manual care.

Turn the usual picture around and consider the therapist's body a mirror image of the effect they are having on the patient. Briefly stated, light contact may be reflected throughout the therapist's body.

It would follow that therapists who use coercive techniques would not have the opportunity to sense the change in them that might accompany a change in the patient. It is hard to hear another when you are shouting at the person.

I have come across patients whom I really did not want to handle much. It was not a matter of hygiene, but rather my sense that their way of being might, in some way, become my own. As I mature, I realize that these people simply represent parts of me that I refuse to acknowledge. If I want to understand myself better, I need to be with people who tend to be the ways that I am not.

Caregivers who gladly take on the patient nobody else wants, the difficult cases, commonly become more authentic, compassionate, and whole.

Henry Blake once described Frank Burns as, "The biggest horse's patoot in the US Army." It sure seemed that way. The hidden benefits of caring for others escaped him. They need not escape us.

Selected Reading

Dorko BL. Manual contact and reflexive effect. *PT Today*. 1989;Winter.

THE DARKENED ROOM

As a PT student trailing behind a therapist in a Columbus hospital, I remember standing at the bedside of an elderly woman, wispy white hair, multiply contractured, unresponsive, breathing with difficulty. The order was for range of motion.

Although I had a tendency, at that age, to stride through most tasks, I felt oddly paralyzed at that moment. My smile, my youth, my personality were not going to help me here. I needed information about therapy and about myself I did not yet have.

The room darkens in my memory, and as I watched the therapist bend to the task, I wanted desperately to leave. I did not know much about manual handling at that time, but I clearly sensed the apparent futility of the work being done. I do not remember if I even touched this woman.

The therapist said nothing. We left, and although I am certain there were other patients that day, that one stayed with me. She still does.

We remember people or events to which we can somehow personally relate. I think I must have seen myself in that hospital bed. It is conceivable that any of us could end up like that despite the efforts of modern medicine. Perhaps it was not the meager effect of therapy as I understood it that upset me so much. Maybe it was the helplessness of the patient to which I felt somehow connected.

Davis describes empathy as a kind of gift given us after the specific interaction related to it has occurred. It is enhanced by our awareness of how, in some way, we are all the same: "...by virtue of the fact that we all breathe, we have the capacity to experience the breathlessness of another person, no matter how different that person appears."

I am guessing when I say that many experiences like mine as a student might drive some therapists toward administrative work. At least, they might weaken their resolve to actually handle others in hopes of helping them. Unless we understand that it is the helplessness of the patient as well as our own that we sense, such work may seem too lonesome a task.

The success of therapy is sometimes difficult to measure or express. Maybe it occurs whenever some human connections are made, connections between therapist and patient and between therapist and self.

I can be in that darkened room with more empathy now that I have been around for awhile. I take with me a line from Rilke's *Letters to a Young Poet:* "Perhaps everything terrible is in its deepest being something helpless that wants help from us."

<u>Selected Reading</u>
Davis CM. What is empathy, and can empathy be taught. *Physical Therapy.* 1990;70(11).

MY RIGHT FOOT

Early in the morning as I dress, I notice it again. I am standing on the lateral aspect of my right foot. I do not mean that my weight is just shifted toward the fifth metatarsal. I mean my ankle is fully inverted and I am resting on the lateral aspect of the bone.

My sole is free.

I am a big guy and this is neither comfortable nor efficient. It is familiar though, and I have learned that this posture means that I am anxious about something. My foot tells me to look into my head for more information.

Feldenkrais defines the unconscious in the simplest possible way by stating that it is "all that is not conscious." This is hard to argue with, but I think it is useful to examine several views of unconscious expression.

Freud viewed the unconscious as a repository of repressed materials. Carl Jung expanded upon this immensely to include the notion that the unconscious contains all that we have ever known and expresses that knowledge in dreams, behavior both subtle and obvious, and our tendency to form or avoid specific relationships. Beyond this, Jung believed that each of us is deeply aware of "archetypes," images that are common across cultures and generations. These are symbols of our inner selves or our sensations of maternity, paternity, childhood, and many other aspects of human experience.

The bodily representation of unconscious processes was especially interesting to the late Milton Erickson, the extraordinarily innovative medical hypnotist. While recovering from polio in his late teens, Erickson sat paralyzed, but observant of his family's small indicators of unconsciously motivated movement. He came to understand that the body in its subtle (and sometimes not so subtle) way would express our true desires or agendas, often in direct opposition to our consciously stated demands.

Erickson used his observational skills and analysis to develop numerous methods of hypnotic induction. He was able to demonstrate that the unconscious was immediately accessible to all of us once we understood its expression in our muscular set and movement. He and Feldenkrais met late in their careers and felt a deep kinship.

I have read recently of a Jungian analyst named Arnold Mindell. In several published texts, he describes the difference between what he calls primary and secondary processes. Primary processes correlate to our conscious awareness and secondary processes to those feelings and motives outside of our usual awareness. Since the latter do not represent our usual selves, or at least the selves we would like the world to see, noticing them may produce an identity crisis. Conflict such as this is symbolically projected to our dreams or our body as muscular patterns and sets.

Mindell describes the unconscious as a river continually flowing through our lives and Jung's archetypes as mere snapshots of that river. We cannot hope to stop the flow or slow it or deny it without paying in some way. The physical manifestations of such a conflict may eventually be an organic pathology of some sort, but this is always preceded by some muscular set. Perhaps, it is the "parasitic" muscular contractions Feldenkrais speaks of, or the armoring of Wilhelm Reich, or the facilitated segments of Irvin Korr.

The implications of this thinking for the therapist who examines posture and assumes that muscular strength or length dictates our shape are obvious. The structure and strength of my right lower leg is fine, but that foot will not behave normally until I discover, confront, and embrace whatever it is that is making me anxious this time. I can hardly look at my patient's posture with less confusion than I do my own. Sometimes, it is enough to make your foot curl.

Suggested Reading

Herbert M. Ecofeminist science and the physiology of the living body. *Somatics.* 1990;7(4).

Mindell A. *River's Way.* London: Rutledge and Kegan Paul Ltd; 1985.

*T*HE PASSIVE VOICE

His name was Richard Maxwell. "Dick" was the patient service coordinator at a rehab center in Columbus, shuffling papers, writing memos, and dealing with the personalities of the patients, families, and staff each day. In 1970 he was a very conservative ex-Marine who actually had an autographed picture taken with Spiro Agnew and Bob Hope on his desk. (I wonder what that would be worth today?)

I was struggling academically and financially, and needed a way of impressing those selecting students for the physical therapy program with a quasi-medical job while paying my rent at the same time.

Dick needed somebody to help him each morning, and we seemed a good match.

I hadn't the slightest idea what it meant to be a quadriplegic, but Dick would teach me. Each morning I would drag myself out of bed at 5:30 a.m., and walk several blocks to the building where Dick both lived and worked. Walking through the darkened hallways, I would occasionally glimpse patients half awake and shuddering with the muscular spasms that greeted them each morning. Moonlight still reminds me of this sight.

I learned from Dick's mother and some of the nurses the rudiments of a bed bath, how to shave someone else's face, how to dress another who had no hand function. From Dick, I learned how to do all he needed without aggravating a sleepy man with a quick temper. He was not my patient; he was my boss. There was nothing I could suggest to alter his routine that he had not been through before in the 7 years since his injury. I had to merge with the small motions of his head, and understand the meaning in his face. Dick actually taught me how to perfectly knot his tie in a windsor. Nothing but perfection was accepted and whatever else might be wrong with my dress these days, no one can find fault with my knot.

During my first few months, I would nap in the afternoons and suddenly waken convinced that I had overslept and left Dick waiting. My roommate would watch me race frantically around the apartment, hyperventilating, and moving like early Jerry Lewis until I realized that this was just another manifestation of the job I had accepted. I never mentioned my fear of failure to Dick. I just managed to show up 7 days a week and apply myself to this task over and over again.

All of the manual care I provided for 3 years was passive range. I was not moving joints their full available range, just far enough to accommodate care. Each day I handled limbs that could not be consciously moved or normally sense their being moved. Still, this part of Dick had a way of being alive that was simply more subtle than my own. Unless moved with a certain care and respect, they would object violently with spasm that would preclude further movement until their voice was heeded.

The skills we acquire in life are not always chosen. They are often the end result of what we had to do in order to get by. If we are lucky, the very skill we inadvertently acquire may help us later on, perhaps even shape a significant portion of our chosen work.

Today, I handle patients in a fashion that reminds me of those mornings with Dick. I understand that the body that is not consciously moved is yet not perfectly still. In a way, unique to itself, it always remains reactive to the intent of our touch. Dick's seemingly passive limbs were always wary of my agenda, and I learned to move him with respect for their unconsciously controlled ability to object. This voice wanted to be asked permission to move, and it safeguarded the dignity of every part, paralyzed or not. I have come to hear this voice in all my patients.

I spoke to Dick recently for the first time in 17 years. He is working, he is married, he coaches a young girls' softball team. We are not very different, really. Among other things, he taught me that my disabilities were just harder to see. I think of that when I waken and see the moonlight.

BEYOND INTUITION

"We become physicians only when we know that which is unnamed, invisible, and immaterial, yet has its effect."

Paracelsus, German physician/mystic, 1493-1541

In my office waiting room I have one of those books full of stereograms. These are the pictures you see in the malls surrounded by a bunch of people staring intently, blocking traffic, and occasionally saying, "Oh! I see it!"

It's not unusual to hear a clinician who practices without an array of measuring devices or intricate protocols described as "intuitive," as in, "Oh, Sue doesn't really know what she's doing, she's just real intuitive."

I read that the ability to see the patterns embedded in a stereogram is dependent upon what ophthalmologists call "decoupling"—the eyes looking through the diagram while your lenses focus on its surface. In the real world you never ordinarily use this capacity.

As a clinician who does not depend heavily on detailed measurements, I know that I am occasionally given credit for being intuitive and it makes me cringe. Not because I'm not using intuition, but because of what it has come to imply.

When I read the description of decoupling and divergence used to explain how stereograms are finally seen, and appreciate how unusual this process is, I know that some real work has been done. In fact, when people claim to be unable to decipher these pictures, you find that their time and attention to the task is sorely lacking.

The intuitive clinician puts forth a real effort. In fact, the Latin root, "intureri," means "to look upon." The sudden knowing of what is happening or how to proceed effectively arises from careful observation over time and is not something that magically appears to someone with a "gift." This is why intuition typically grows with experience, as long as the therapist pays attention.

There's a great line from Lewis Carroll specifically about this: "You're not paying Attention," said the Hatter. "If you don't pay him, you know, he won't perform."

I have wondered for some time how the sudden vision of the image in a stereogram after work, time, and attention differs from what I suddenly realize in the clinic and I think I've found it in the quote from Paracelsus at the beginning of this essay.

In addition to what we can sense, name, and measure are processes inaccessible to our most careful scrutiny. We know they are present and we understand their effect only by going to the texts of biophysics, physiology, and pathology designed for our profession. There are plenty.

Without understanding the invisible, we are easily misled and properly thought of as no more skillful than bodyworkers with less education.

Intuition alone may provide my patients with enough to see those pictures in my waiting room, but they need a therapist with even more, and I deserve credit for that, too.

GOING HOME

I live just 45 miles from my boyhood home and my parents still reside there. The airport is near and I often stop on my way to some other state to teach. My father fixes me something to eat and I spend time sitting quietly with my mother.

I know that many people my age don't have this luxury and I treasure it.

Although my aging seems to have made me a good deal wiser and more patient, I can see and feel that my body isn't what it once was and since I often work with Medicare-eligible patients, I am very familiar with what it may become.

Thomas Moore points out that the Greek root of the word ecology is "oikos," meaning "home." He feels that when we gain a sense of at-homeness in our environment, we will quite naturally treat it with care and respect.

At my age the changes creeping through me often have the kind of numerical values that our profession thrives on. I hate them.

Being at home with my parents still comes easily to me. Despite the fact that my personal dimensions have dramatically changed since childhood, everything from the furniture to the utensils still fit comfortably. I can't seem to outgrow this feeling. In my home environment I always find a way of being that is healthy in a variety of ways.

I wonder how I would feel here if one day I was told by someone in authority that this home was poorly decorated, that it was in need of a new coat of paint, not because the old one was gone, but just because somebody else didn't like the shade. Could I remain comfortable at home in the face of a media barrage of alternatives that were touted as healthier and more impressive to others?

I don't need a mirror to tell me what age is doing, I can feel it pretty well. I'm hopeful that I can maintain an attitude that reminds me to attend to things beyond the cosmetic. Sometimes I see patients who have somehow maintained their health while becoming indifferent to mirrors, and I admire that.

I've come to feel that these people have chosen an "ecology of the body." They are comfortable with the naturally occurring change in their shape and have learned that health is something felt on the inside more than displayed on the surface.

In the second half of their life they feel at home with what they have. They find nurturance and acceptance within their own systems, and major redecorating is of no interest.

One day these trips to my boyhood home will stop. I'd better bring some of that feeling out into the world with me.

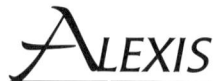LEXIS

Alexis joined our staff just about a month ago. She's still here part-time, but we're hoping to increase her hours in the near future.

This is a small office and each of us makes an impact. It's always interesting to watch the changes each new person brings with them. I've seen each of us here trying to adjust to a new seating arrangement, a change in our space for paperwork, and a decrease in our share of attention and time to talk now that there is somebody else to listen to.

I stress the quality of acceptance to my staff and patients. I tell them that I have learned many times that to approach every situation without judgment is the best way to see it with clarity. I strive to choose acceptance when I listen to patients and when I touch them. I talk a lot about how acceptance of another person or situation does not imply resignation to the status quo. In fact, acceptance immediately precedes change. This is just as true of interpersonal relations as it is of backache. Sometimes I go on to speak of how all of this begins with self-acceptance, which is perhaps the hardest thing to learn.

I should add here that I regularly serve as a perfect example of what judgment can do to make us unhappy. Sometimes I even judge my own body, and it becomes increasingly rigid in response. Pain eventually comes and I'm driven to return to acceptance once again. It's obvious that knowing all of this does not save me from years of acting otherwise. Acceptance is a new road for me.

Somehow it appears that Alexis does not need any of my lofty lectures. I have yet to see her approach any situation or person with anything other than genuine openness and immediate interest. She is truly intimate with everything and everyone here. Described by Malone and Malone, "Intimacy is the quality of becoming more yourself while in relation to something else." Alexis is so completely authentic with all of us and every patient, that I seem stiff in comparison.

Sometimes I lecture my classes on how manual care should include attention to the ever-changing relationship the therapist has with the patient. As our hands monitor and affect change, I am altered, and there is much to be learned from this. It is clear that Alexis already knows all that.

There is one more thing—her hands. One of my favorite short stories is "Neighbor Rosicky" by Willa Cather. Rosicky is an old farmer in Nebraska who displays the same acceptance, sensitivity, and joyful embrace of living that I see in Alexis. His hands are described in detail by Cather as: "warm and human, flexible and nimble, generous and lively. Not like other farmers: a huge lump of fist with stiff fingers. [You could] never learn so much about life from anything as from old Rosicky's hand. It brings you to yourself, and communicates some direct and untranslatable message."

Alexis has those same hands and often stares into them as if trying to learn more. I wish I had those hands.

Of course, Alexis is just 2 months old and the first daughter of my long-time partner Jennifer Gable. She has changed the way we are around here. Sometimes we tiptoe, and we certainly smile more. Beyond that, we are reminded of how we all once were and would like to be again.

Selected Reading

Cather W. Neighbor Rosicky. *Great Short Works of Willa Cather*. New York, NY: Perennial Library; 1960.

Malone T, Malone P. *The Art of Intimacy*. New York, NY: Prentice Hall; 1987.

CETTING ARRESTED

"Someone must have been telling lies about Joseph K., for without having done anything wrong he was arrested one fine morning."

Franz Kafka, from *The Trial*

This somewhat startling sentence begins Kafka's classic novel about a man caught up in a bizarre and compelling circumstance. He finds himself quite unexpectedly accused of an unnamed offense by a seemingly faceless and random bureaucracy. His frantic attempts to resolve this conflict expose both the corrupt attributes of those in authority and K.'s own emotional barrenness.

The analyst Erich Fromm argues that this novel must be understood as a dream "...[where] each event is itself concrete and realistic; yet the whole is impossible and fantastic."

Fromm points out that although the term "arrested" as manifest in Kafka's story would ordinarily be something that disrupts the normal day to day living of one's life; Joseph K. is not made to alter his normal routine of work. Fromm feels that the word arrested must instead mean that the man is stunted or allowed not to grow. Kafka's brief description of the whole of Joseph K.'s ordinary routine (one paragraph) makes it clear that this man is an impersonal receiver of life and the services he can afford. He offers nothing to others.

Do you ever feel "arrested?" Are there times when the routine of running a practice designed to support you and your staff and your dependents and their dependents makes you wish that you saw more patients who could be placed on a kind of conveyor belt, treated generically, and billed as they came off?

As I travel and teach, I often hear from therapists claiming to be tired of seeing chronic patients who are "all the same." Of course, this can only be true in the mind of the therapist. I think that there is only one way to make all your patients look alike—treat them all the same.

Practicing like this might be one way of making a living, but it is also guaranteed to produce an "arrest" of your growth as a therapist.

You may begin to feel less of the art that the innovators in physical therapy have always displayed as the consequence of their fresh vision of each patient they encounter. To the best clinicians, subtle differences between patients are not only obvious but extremely important. If the manner in which our patients gesture, posture, and finally structure themselves is our primary concern, it is obvious that they couldn't all look the same. Perhaps this would be somewhat possible if we only considered one body part (e.g., their knees) and only then if our view just included the orthopedic elements with no thought of their connections to a unique central nervous system. Of course, no living body actually exists this way. Pretending that it does produces repetitive, generic, ineffective care and an arrested therapist.

What can be done to avoid this phenomena when the patients come in droves and instituting protocols for diagnoses seems so financially expedient? The answer is not easy, but it is clearly implied by Kafka and discussed by Fromm. Joseph K.'s arrest was the end result of his nature. His inability to obtain release was the end result of his view of authority.

I doubt that many of us went into our profession with the attitude that we would not give to others. However, our view of authority may at times interfere with our own personal liberation from arrested growth.

Joseph K. could see no distinction between civil authority and his own conscience as represented initially by an inspector who says "...think less about us and of what is to happen to you; think more about yourself instead." Later, K. is confronted dramatically by a priest. "You cast about too much for outside help...don't you see that it isn't the right kind of help?" The priest also makes this point: "The Court makes no claims upon you. It receives you when you come and it relinquishes you when you go." This view is the opposite of authoritarianism.

K. is offered the opportunity to find a way of escaping his arrest by looking inside himself, by having some faith in his own feelings, shaped by his experience and knowledge and not dictated by some outside authority. His inability to do this results ultimately in his execution.

The therapists who feel arrested in their growth as clinicians often try to fix this by racing frantically from course to course as time and finances allow. They look for answers from authorities. In my experience this will never produce any real growth unless there is a simultaneous inward questioning of the therapist's original motivation and a continued awareness of one's own unique perceptual ability. If the therapist truly attends to his or her patient's experience of their problem, they may being to see that while authorities may offer some insight, real growth occurs when the therapist takes personal responsibility for learning from his or her own experience. The therapist must acquire an intuitive knowledge of each patient that arises from the actual observation of that patient's unique presentation. Recall that the word intuition comes from the Latin "intuere" meaning "to look upon."

Kafka's novels contain darkness, confusion, absurdity, and anxiety. Sounds like my practice at times in the past. There is, however, a persistent element of the tenacious longing for meaning that all humans share.

We can only avoid arrest by remaining vigilant of our motives and ensuring that the giving side of our practice does not exceed the taking. If arrested, the only true path toward extrication and growth begins within ourselves.

<u>Selected Reading</u>
Fromm E. *The Forgotten Language*. New York, NY: Rinehart and Co, Inc; 1951.
Kafka F. *The Trial*. New York, NY: Alfred Knopf; 1960.

Without Them

I am not and will not soon become a therapist that the medical community can relate to. I have struggled with this as long as I can remember and see no end in sight.

Perhaps I do not belong in the company of physicians simply because we have two remarkably different perspectives of the same patient. This would not ordinarily be a problem, but when our interpretation of the patient's function and feeling do not match, one of us must yield, and I carry no expertise into this discussion that many physicians will honor. When the battleground is the patient's body, I would much prefer not to raise my voice in anger although I know that I have.

$\mathcal{N}_o$

Get this, I recently had sent to my office a proposed prescription form for physical therapy from a young orthopedist in my area. He had recently complained to my partner that other therapists in our town had not been "following my orders" when sent a patient with a specific diagnosis. They had not strictly adhered to the protocols for care provided by his office and (this was the worst) they had actually evaluated the patient prior to care.

The surgeon was incensed, but he felt that he might have hit upon a solution. He put together a prescription form for "spine problems," another for "knee problems," and a third for "shoulder problems." Each form had a brief list of potential diagnoses with space for a check mark, followed by a list of possible instructions for the therapist, each with another space to check. The form is simplicity itself: compact, clear, easily read.

By now I'm sure many of you are shaking your heads and smiling. I mean smiling ruefully. In fact, I know therapists have seen even more restrictive orders from their referral sources. But there's more.

Beneath "follow protocol" is another option this physician can check. It says "NO evaluation necessary." Notice the "O" is capitalized. I guess this is so the therapist won't miss that word. I suppose the doctor wants to make it clear that just a little evaluation will not be tolerated; he means none at all. There is a note accompanying these forms, "Please review and share your comments. What do you know about the physical therapy practice act? Do all PTs need to evaluate prior to prescribed PT?" (The doctor underlined "all" himself.)

My good friend Sam Kegerreis teaches at the University of Indianapolis and treats patients in a private office. He tells a story about his first introduction to a patient with a chronic and severe shoulder problem. This man had trouble with his employer, his family, you name it. What struck Sam most when he first saw him though was the man's dress. He was sitting in the waiting room in a Goofy hat. The kind with a nose on the bill, eyes on the crown, and those long back ears that hang down to your neck. Remember, this is Indiana, not Orlando. Sam says, "This was my patient. This is what I had to work with."

Sometimes in this business you are presented with a situation that seems overwhelming in its scope and complexity. It is hard to imagine how some things come to be and our only hope is to live with the people in this event and try to understand their perspective and motivations.

Sam Kegerreis, being the therapist he is, attended carefully to the man in the Goofy hat. My guess is that he might have even (gasp) evaluated him. Sam came to understand his patient's perspective and motivation. The therapist and patient came together and both benefited. The patient returned to work and Sam has a great story to tell.

I feel as if the surgeon that would prefer NO evaluation is as far from my way of seeing the PT's role as he could possibly be. The man in the hat would be easier to connect with. At least he and I have similar goals. I'm not so sure about the doctor.

How does a surgeon get to this point? How can I help him without speaking in a manner he would find offensive?

This is tough. It seems clear that the doctor is not looking for help, but rather for more control. I don't think he wants a discussion, and maybe all that I can say is contained in the title of this essay. Of course, he said it first and just now it looks like nobody will benefit.

PREFERENCES

Sitting at lunch with two orthopedists a few years ago, I had a conversation I have thought of many times since.

I wondered aloud how you could possibly touch someone's head and produce a sensation in their feet.

One doctor spoke of the various nerves that would require depolarization. We discussed the possible modes of energy transmission that might make it possible for stimulation in one area to lead to sensation, change, or movement elsewhere. We considered the contribution of sensory input not previously thought of.

The other doctor listened absently for a while and then interrupted.

"You touch their heads and they say that they feel it in their feet?"

"Yes."

"Patient's crazy."

End of discussion.

I wanted to say, "Gee, I hadn't thought of that! Here all this time I just assumed that several thousand people in my office were authentically expressing what they felt. To think that they were all just 'crazy'...Thanks, Doc!

I wanted to say, "What makes you think you can immediately dismiss my clinical observations as if I were no more than a candy-striper?"

I wanted to say, "How would you know? The only time you ever really express an interest in patients is when they are anesthetized."

I wanted to say, "Is there something about me that you deny so strongly in yourself that my mere presence elicits an immediate negative reaction?" (This is a rather esoteric psychological ploy he probably would not have understood.)

Of course, I didn't say anything. I just went back to eating.

What is it that so often produces an enormous gulf between therapists and physicians? For me, it has been a gulf full of fear, anger, frustration, worry, and resentment.

In *Gathering Power* by Ken Keyes, these are described as "separating emotions" and are the consequence of the demands I have made on my environment and of the people around me. If this is the case, I have to ask, "What do I demand of physicians?"

Well, I demand that they respect my knowledge and skills. It is a fact, however, that most of my referral sources have never seen or spoken to me and express little interest in doing so.

Demands by definition cannot be met and they imply that if what I demand does not happen soon I must act. My action begins with anger and fear and things worsen from that point on.

Keyes suggests we upgrade our demands to preferences. Preferences can include all of the things we used to demand but do not carry the baggage of negative emotion. Preferences always remain despite the actions of others. If I wait long enough, things might always work out the way I had hoped.

I know that I should have preferred that this doctor listen. I should have preferred that he show some respect for my patients and my experience. Lunch would have been easier to eat, and although the gulf between us might have remained, it wouldn't have been filled with all the bad stuff I normally felt there.

Since that time I have learned how a certain technique at the head might be felt in the foot. It's the subject of the essay "Tsunami." It doesn't have anything to do with my patients being crazy. I hope that that orthopedist reads it. But, he doesn't have to.

Selected Reading
Keyes K. *Gathering Power.* Coos Bay, Ore: Living Love Press; 1987.

BACK TO THE BEGINNING

In 1975, I was among just four therapists who had completed all of Stan Paris's courses in spinal and extremity manipulation. (There were only three courses in his curriculum at the time.) On the strength of this, plus a series of misunderstandings and coincidences, I became the Senior Clinician at the Atlanta Back Clinic when it first opened.

I was 24, had struggled mightily to get through school, and had spent the previous year doing range of motion and gait training in several different nursing homes. Of course, this didn't keep me from having a lot of opinions about just exactly what should be done for people with spinal pain. When Stan left to teach, I was alone and because of my title, many people looked to me for advice and the manual handling at which I was supposed to be expert. Looking back at this always makes me shake my head.

In *The Heart Aroused*, David Whyte writes of how, after obtaining a degree in marine biology, he was hired as a guide in the Galapagos Islands. Whyte points out that for people in his profession, this was the best job you could possibly get; equivalent, he says, to becoming the "greatest poet in Ireland."

In 1975 I had a similar position. Therapists interested in manual care at that time had little freedom to practice as they wished and no regular access to the originators of theory and technique. I was surrounded by this.

After a few weeks in the Galapagos, Whyte realized that "The animals had apparently not read the same books that I had." I can remember noticing the same thing about my patients in Atlanta. On top of that, some of them seemed totally unimpressed with my remarkable skills and vast store of knowledge.

I couldn't believe it.

Yesterday I saw another new patient. Her orthopedist handed her a list of therapy offices in the Akron area and mine happened to be near her home. She found that parking next to my building was easy as well, so she picked me to see. Her doctor made it clear that he had absolutely no interest in who she was going to see. He thinks therapists are as alike as pharmacists.

While in Atlanta I worked daily beside Bob Donatelli, Steve Krause,

Rich Nyberg, and Mariano Rocabado. I traveled and taught with Paris, Ola Grimsby, John Mennell, and Freddy Kaltenborn. I spent time in the clinic with Cliff Fowler, one of the founders of Canadian manual therapy training and the best clinician I've ever met. All of these men have personally shaped the way orthopedic care is practiced in North America, and they taught me directly.

Does the patient care about the years I've spent in the company of therapists who really know what they're doing? I've watched countless evaluative and treatment techniques develop, endure, disappear, resurface, and disappear again. Referral sources who care about that I can count on one hand.

Each day, at least for awhile, I feel much as I did in Atlanta 20 years ago. I don't know much about what might be wrong. I'm unsure about what to do next and the patients often act toward me as the animals did toward David Whyte—they aren't impressed by my credentials, and they are what they are. And unpredictably that.

Each day I begin again, just me and the patient with nothing between us but what we think we know, and what we are about to learn.

Selected Reading

Whyte D. *The Heart Aroused*. New York, NY: Doubleday; 1994.

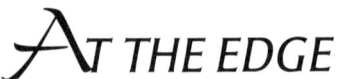# AT THE EDGE

"Come to the edge", he said.
We might fall
It's too high!
"COME TO THE EDGE"
So they came
And he pushed
And they flew

Christopher Logue

There have been moments in my career when what I felt to be a forward movement in my skills and knowledge was resisted in some way. I sensed this resistance in the attitudes of my co-workers, my superiors, and my patients when I tried to explain some new idea about the nature of disability and what some therapy might accomplish (these were usually someone else's ideas and I had just returned from another workshop).

Although the long-term effect of my new knowledge varied greatly, the resistance I encountered was always pretty much the same at first. My passion for some new technique rarely swayed other therapists with long-established patterns of perception and valid reasons of their own for proceeding with the same, safe protocols as always.

I realize now that my enthusiasm for change was connected to my fascination for the "edge" of clinical practice. In a recent essay by Catherine Peck, the edge is described as a place full of creative activity and conflict. Like any border, it is a place of transition, and resistance to our movement across it is to be expected. At this border, we naturally work to find some order in the chaos of a new frontier. If accepted and proven methods of treatment resemble a civilized and lawful country, our step to the edge may alternately be into a place where all the rules are not yet know.

Only after living here for some time will we learn how to measure things reliably. At the edge, provocation may elicit an unexpected response and protocols are not yet set.

When we discover the rules that new procedures follow we may see their worth and validity. In fact, if no consistent response to a new method emerges, we must begin to wonder if we are on the threshold of a useful procedure or just taking a walk on the wild side. In retrospect, ineffective care simply combines the best of intentions with the worst of ideas.

When practicing on the edge becomes increasingly chaotic, when theory defies physical law, or when the specter of placebo cannot be dispelled, it is time to let go and return home.

Sometimes when we sense an edge or border approaching we resent it. It represents limits, and if we feel that we can somehow accomplish whatever we want with enough effort, the resistance inevitable at the edge may invite attack. A therapist with a new idea might self-righteously say, "They laughed at Fulton, they laughed at Edison."

The problem with that argument is that they also laughed at Bozo the Clown.

Over the years I have watched new ideas rise, become accepted, and flourish (TENS, manipulation, isokinetics). I have watched others wither (Applied Kinesiology, Inversion Therapy). Today, cranial work balances on the edge and I'm there once again.

Fortunately, rules and reasonable theory are becoming evident. If I don't strike out at the resistance, if I remain vigilant for movement forward that makes sense, the edge will remain before me and I won't fall, I'll fly.

Selected Reading
Peck C. Reflections on the edge. *The Yoga Journal.* 1991;Sept/Oct.

Rust Out

I want to mow lawns for a living. I am perfectly serious about this. Yesterday, through a window in my office, I watched as some crew member of the firm I pay to maintain the grounds walked back and forth with the mower and it sure looked like a good job to me. I know something about this because I spent two summers in my youth doing the same thing. I remember that there was a wonderful, steady rhythm to the striding I would do behind the mower. Finishing each lawn, lifting the equipment, and riding in the truck to the next job provided another rhythm that I found remarkably satisfying.

When you mow lawns for a living, nature is your referral source. Every week it sends more work your way and it always forgives you for failing to perform a miracle on the last lawn. Nature never asks you for part of the money you earn just because it made the grass grow. Nature does not suddenly stop sending you lawns to mow for no apparent reason. Nature never accuses you of being weird just because you approach lawn mowing in a nontraditional way. Nature holds no grudges because it thinks you have a mind of your own and it never expects you to mow its relatives for free.

If I mowed lawns for a living, I would probably never run into a massive bureaucracy that whimsically denied payment for work already done. No agency would set limits on the number of mowings allowed despite the fact that the grass continued to grow. I would not be asked to mow grass that did not need it and when a job was completed everyone would agree that it was so.

As a member of the crew, I would not have to worry about staffing, regulations, inspections by Medicare, or earning continuing education credits. I would probably be able to keep up with the advancements in the industry just by doing what the boss told me to do.

Therapists are often described as individuals driven by the caregiver within them. But sometimes the heavy load of administration and the capricious nature of marketing can overwhelm the part of us that led us into the profession to begin with. In the bestseller *Fire in the Belly*, Sam Keen suggests that many of us suffer not from burnout, but rust out. Rust out happens when the fire and the passion with which we begin our lives is stifled by the circumstances that ask for something else, something that was not part of our original intent.

I still care, but some days I honestly feel that lawn care would be enough.

Selected Reading

Keen S. *Fire in the Belly.* New York, NY: Bantam; 1991.

A FINE, ICY DAY

There was a fine, icy day here in early February. Like many others, Valerie fell, landed on her sacrum, and found that she could not do her job that day or the next. She went to her family physician and he ordered 2 weeks of bedrest.

A few weeks ago, I flew to Houston where a secretary from the practice sponsoring my workshop was to meet me at the curb outside baggage claim. She had my photo. My flight was delayed and when I finally stepped to the curb a dozen people in as many cars looked directly at me without recognition and I wandered up and down, thinking about how much I enjoy this part of traveling.

Valerie felt worse after 2 weeks off work and her doctor sent her to see an orthopedist in the building next to mine. He said "No fracture, only a contusion. You'll have to wait 2 months."

It was cold and windy on that curb in Houston and after a while, I went inside to call the practice. "We know she's there. She called to tell us you would be arriving late." I had the secretary paged.

Valerie grew worse still. The family physician's office called and arranged an appointment with me. Her history and exam did not reveal anything that I felt couldn't be easily helped and in three visits she was ready and willing to return to work. It was now mid-April.

I walked back to the curb at the airport and heard the call for my ride to meet me there. Ten feet away a lady looked up immediately, surprised to see me standing where I had been for half an hour.

Valerie has been 2 weeks back to work and says she actually feels better than before she fell. The family physician is fully aware of her recovery. In the 10 years he has sent patients to me, he has seen similar responses the four or five times each year that he orders therapy from his large practice. Most of his patients wonder aloud about the delay in their care.

The orthopedist hasn't a clue what happened. We've had a few mutual patients and I successfully treated his wife a few years ago. Each Christmas I get invited to his party. I know that his ability to assess and manage a surgical candidate is excellent.

My ride in Houston explained to me that she had been told my plane wouldn't land for another hour. It was clear that she couldn't and didn't see me for a simple reason—I wasn't supposed to be there.

I know that many therapists think their referral sources are unreliable because they refuse to be educated about the benefits of therapy. Therapists know that some doctors need a financial incentive, that others are just jealous of our skills or feel they are only palliative.

Maybe the two doctors Valerie and I recently worked with are just unable to see something because they don't know it could possibly be there. Although I'm sure some marketing people would disagree, I don't think this can be fixed. I've tried "paging" these men for years.

I think the referral for a patient like this is actually something aside from the medical community. It comes naturally to every practice and doesn't discriminate between those in managed care or with traditional insurance coverage. It treats all levels of society, age groups, and both genders alike and isn't blinded by the notion that something is not "supposed" to be there. It jolts the patient toward my office despite the doctor.

It is that fine, icy day.

The CONSULTATION

In a few moments he will cut open the lateral aspect of this woman's left thigh and inspect the tissue to determine how he might proceed with the repair of the bone. He hasn't actually seen the x-ray or the report yet, but he has heard that it's a day-old subcapital fracture and right now he thinks a bipolar arthroplasty will be sufficient. He tells the nurse he wants the x-rays.

Her husband of 56 years and her youngest son stand together at the head of the bed and he states his name. Well, not his whole name. Just "Dr." and the last name. After the son reaches for his hand and introduces himself, he wants to begin his preop spiel but stops short when forced to meet the older man as well.

After his succinct statement of protocol for aftercare for such a procedure, including an admonition not to cross her legs and some period of recovery in an extended care facility, he is told by the son that this broken hip belongs to a woman who has severe Alzheimer's.

There is just the barest pause in the pace of his delivery. Although it could not be said that his expression softens, he begins to think of what this new information implies and in his eyes the son sees that the options of recovery have narrowed. Suddenly the procedure he is about to perform is less likely to help in the usual way, because the hip is now attached to something he can't control.

There is a small space of silence as he considers this, and the son interrupts again to tell him that his mother spent many years in the presence of one of his partners as a nurse on an orthopedic ward. The husband tells him that that is why we chose him to do this today, because his older colleague was often mentioned at dinner.

All of this seems a good deal more about the fracture than he needs to know, and the white-haired, wheezened woman with eyes closed, labored breathing beneath the blanket is now actually starting to stir and wince. Her son sees the middle-aged nurse who used to stand quietly by such a doctor, patiently listening and diligently performing the tasks of care she now so desperately needs from him. He is trying to offer the doctor this vision, coaxing the words from a tight throat full of so much more.

It seems too much. There isn't time. He needs the x-ray now. He barely hears the husband say something more about this hip on the bed and some internal gate he uses to shut out this kind of information closes barely in time. It is too late to stifle the tearful inflection of the old man's voice, the same awful sound he just heard from the son.

He's a man of action, broad-chested and narrow at the waist. He acts now. Enough talk. Already too much time. Despite his size the handshake is limp, and very fast, and the eyes are elsewhere. He is off to where he doesn't have to hear any more voices like this.

And the son wonders how a man comes to be like this. And what he can do to escape it himself. And he turns to his father and sees how different the doctor could be, if only he knew what he had just done.

ALONE

I work with patients with a primary complaint of spinal pain, and often it's not a job I would wish on anybody.

I wouldn't say that it is necessarily more demanding or requires more skill or knowledge than many other specialties. I'm not even sure it's a specialty, in any strict sense, although I think that many therapists, and most physicians, would rather this complaint not clog up their schedules as it tends to. Its presence disrupts any practice that depends upon protocols, clear diagnoses, and predictable responses to care. It is a specialty in that it is especially irritating to so many caregivers.

A recent article by Karel Lewit cites 20 characteristics of functional and/or pathologic diagnostics and treatment, and, as far as I'm concerned, it says more, sensibly, about spinal complaints than all the "categorizations" of this problem I have ever seen.

Lewit doesn't offer a flow chart to assist in management and he doesn't begin by citing the enormous cost of backache in dollars and days lost from work. In fact, he doesn't mention spinal pain at all. It just sounds like it when he lists the characteristics of dysfunction and its treatment.

For example:

"Whoever only treats dysfunction at the point where pain is felt is lost, or rather, his patient is lost."

"...if the dysfunction is adequately treated (and the case is not very complicated), the effect of the treatment is immediate, giving the impression of a 'miracle cure'; which, however, is quite predictable."

"The functional approach is much more difficult. We may compare pathology to the 'hardware' and dysfunction to the 'software' of the motor system."

I want to emphasize that Lewit's brief article shows him to be a clinician with a great deal of respect for what his patient brings with him to care. He doesn't begin with a bias but an appreciation for the complexity of human functioning and its ability to save us from symptoms when pathology strikes. He also knows that dysfunction in the absence of any anatomical abnormality can hurt, and, in my experience, this is not common knowledge.

The Greek work "idiopatheia" means "a feeling for oneself alone" or "suffering for oneself." It is the origin of "idiopathic," and people with that word in their diagnoses can relate to the isolation they may feel as the experts shrug their shoulders when asked to explain the origins or perpetuation of their complaint.

I don't know that any single complaint of pain is more likely to produce a shrug, a raised eyebrow, or a confusion of care than spinal pain. One local referral source always circles both "Williams" (emphasize flexion) and "McKenzie" (emphasize extension) on his own prescription pad for therapy.

It stands to reason that those of us who have chosen to spend each day with these patients often feel we're practicing a kind of idiopathic therapy—alone, poorly understood, frustrating, and mysterious.

Lewit's article helps. I just wish somebody would read it.

Selected Reading
Lewit K. The functional approach. *The Journal of Orthopaedic Medicine*. 1994;16(3).

THE LAST RESORT

"Well, you're really not progressing as I had hoped and it looks like I'm going to have to send you to a therapist in the Falls."

"What's so special about this guy?"

"I'm not sure really, and I've never actually spoken to him. But every once in a while I send him a real tough case like yours and most of them report that they did really well."

"He's not going to dig his knuckles into my neck like that last therapist, is he? I thought I was going to die for several hours after each visit."

"Oh no, I understand his handling is very gentle, and I've never heard anyone complain that they were hurt or asked to do anything that increased their pain."

"Well then, just what exactly does he do?"

"Let's see, I have a letter here from him. He sent it after he treated last year's patient. He says, 'Although this patient displays no frank neurological signs, the persistent sympathetic dominance that has accompanied all of her symptoms might be an indication of adverse neural tension. This would account for her pain, the coolness of her limbs, her difficulty with normal sleep, her upper respiratory breathing pattern, and her increase in symptoms after prolonged positioning. A problem such as this will often worsen in response to traditional exercise regimes designed to strengthen or stretch the body.'"

"I didn't understand all of that but it sure sounded like he was describing me and how I felt after doing what I was told. And his office is 10 minutes from here."

"Yes, I agree, and that is why I want you to go and see this guy, here's his number."

"Are you going to call him before I get there?"

"I hadn't planned on it."

"How's he going to know what's wrong with me? How's he going to know what to do? You told the last therapist what to do."

"Yes, well...this guy does something different and I'm not really sure he wants me to write an order. Like I said, I use him for really tough cases like yours."

"How come you waited for a year before deciding to try something else for me? I told you 6 months ago how badly I was doing. Wasn't that long enough to wait before sending me to someone who wasn't going to hurt me and understood all my complaints?"

"Look, why don't you just give this guy a call and see if he can't help you. In the meantime I don't want you to make anymore appointments with me. Maybe just give me a call if you don't get any better."

"So this is it? You're getting rid of me?"

"I'm sending you to a specialist. I'm hopeful that he can help."

"But you don't know what he does, and, you've never spoken to him, and you don't plan on discussing my condition with him before I get there."

"Well, that's all true."

"Thanks a lot. I guess if I get better, I won't see you."

SELECTED READING

Ackerman D. *A Natural History of the Senses*. New York, NY: Vintage Books; 1991.

Bennett R. Does fibrositis exist and can it be treated? *Journal of Musculoskeletal Medicine*. 1984;1(7).

Berman M. *Coming to Our Senses*. New York, NY: Simon & Schuster; 1989.

Bly R. My father's wedding. *The Man in the Black Coat Turns*. New York, NY: Dial Press; 1981.

Breig A, Troup J. Biomechanical considerations in the straight-leg-raising test. *Spine*. 1979;4(3).

Briggs J, Monaco R. *Metaphor: The Logic of Poetry*. New York, NY: Pace University Press; 1990.

Brooks C. *Sensory Awareness: The Rediscovery of Experiencing*. Santa Barbara, Calif: Ross-Erikson; 1974.

Butler D. *Mobilisation of the Nervous System*. Melbourne: Churchill Livingstone; 1991.

Cather W. Neighbor Rosicky. *Great Short Works of Willa Cather*. New York, NY: Perennial Library; 1960.

Cyriax J. *Textbook of Orthopaedic Medicine*. Vol 1. Baltimore, Md: Williams & Wilkins: 73.

Davis CM. What is empathy, and can empathy be taught. *Physical Therapy*. 1990;70(11).

Donaldson OF. Play to win and every victory is a funeral. *Somatics*. 1984;4(4).

Donaldson OF. *Playing By Heart*. Deerfield Beach, Fla: Health Communications Inc; 1993.

Dorko BL. Adaptive potential: a new concept in pain of mechanical origin. *PT Forum*. 1988;7(29).

Dorko BL. Juggling philosophically. *Jugglers World*. 1989;Spring.

Dorko BL. Manual contact and reflexive effect. *PT Today*. 1989;Winter.

Dorko BL. Perceptual clarity in PT. *PT Bulletin*. 1989;Apr 12.

Dorko BL. Simple Contact and Distant Change. Unpublished copies available from the author.

Dorland's Medical Dictionary. 27th ed. Philadelphia, Pa: WB Saunders; 1988.

Duff K. *The Alchemy of Illness*. New York, NY: Pantheon; 1993.

Dwinell M. My father. *The Best of Pilgrimage*. Vol 1. 1986-1992.

Edelman G. *Neural Darwinism*. New York, NY: Basic Books; 1987.

Elmer-Dewit P. Reliving polio. *Time*. 1994;Mar 28.

Estes. *Sounds True Catalogue*. 1993;Feb.

Feil N. Validation therapy. *Somatics*. 1991-1992;8(3).

Feldenkrais M. *The Elusive Obvious*. Cupertino, Calif: Meta Publications; 1981.

Fiser K. *Words Like Fate and Pain*. Cambridge, Mass: Zoland Books; 1992.

Fisher A. *The Essential Writings of Merleau-Ponty*. New York, NY: Harcourt Brace; 1969.

Frank A. *At the Will of the Body*. Boston, Mass: Houghton Mifflin; 1991.

Fromm E. *The Forgotten Language*. New York, NY: Rinehart and Co, Inc; 1951.

Gellhorn E. *Somatic-Automatic Integrations: Physiologic Basis and Clinical Implications*. Minneapolis, Minn: University of Minnesota Press; 1967.

Glashow S. Tangled in supersting. *The Sciences*. 1988;May/Jun.

Goldberg N. *Wild Mind: Living the Writer's Life*. New York, NY: Bantam; 1990.

Goldberger A, Rigney D, West B. Chaos and fractals in human physiology. *Scientific American*. 1990;Feb.

Goldsmith. Chaos: to see a world in a grain of sand and heaven in a wild flower. *Archives of Dermatology*. 1990;Sept.

Gould J. The art of physical therapy. *SOSPT*. 1990;Feb. Editorial.

Grandin T, Scariano. *Emergence: Labeled Autistic*. Arena Press; 1986.

Grieve GP. Scrutinizing tacit assumptions in manual therapy. *Journal of Manual and Manipulative Therapy*. 1993;1(4).

Guharay, Sachs F. Stretch-activated single ion channel currents in tissue-cultured embryonic chick skeletal muscle. *Journal of Physiology*. 1984;352:685-701.

Hanna T. What is somatics? *Somatics*. 1986;5(4).

Harrington D. Body of faith. *The Humanistic Psychologist*. 1987;15.

Heckler RS. A holy curiosity. *Somatics*. 1990-1991;Autumn/Winter.

Heelan PA. *Space Perception and the Philosophy of Science*. Berkeley, Calif: University of California Press; 1983.

Herrigel E. *Zen in the Art of Archery*. New York, NY: Vintage Books; 1971.

Hillman J, Ventura M. *We've Had One Hundred Years of Psychotherapy and the World Is Getting Worse*. San Francisco, Calif: Harper; 1992.

Huang A. *Embrace Tiger, Return to Mountain—The Essence of T'ai Chi*. Moab, Utah: Real People Press; 1973.

I'm not handicapped in my brain. *Clinical Management*. 1992;12(3).

Jensen GM. Qualitative methods in physical therapy research: a form of disciplined injury. *Physical Therapy*. 1989;69(6).

Johnson D. Somatic platonism. *Somatics*. 1980;3(1).

Johnson DH. *Body, Spirit and Democracy*. Berkeley, Calif: North Atlantic Books; 1994.

Johnson DH. Principles versus techniques. *Somatics*. 1986;Autumn/Winter.

Johnson R. *Owning Your Own Shadow*. San Francisco, Calif: Harper Collins; 1991.

Kafka F. *The Trial*. New York, NY: Alfred Knopf; 1960.

Keen S. *Fire in the Belly*. New York, NY: Bantam; 1991.

Keen S, Valley-Fox A. *Your Mythic Journey*. Los Angeles, Calif: Tarcher; 1989.

Kendall F. Catherine Worthingham Fellow Forum; Cincinnati, Ohio; June 1993.

Keyes K. *Gathering Power*. Coos Bay, Ore: Living Love Press; 1987.

Korr I. *The Neurobiologic Mechanisms in Manipulative Therapy*. New York, NY: Plenum Press; 1978.

Korr I. Symposium on the functional implications of segmental facilitation. *JOAO*. 1955;54(5).

Kostopoulous DC, Keramidas G. Changes in elongation of falx cerebri during cran-iosacral therapy techniques applied on the skull of an embalmed cadaver. *J Craniomandibular Practice*. 1992;10(1).

Kostopoulous DC, Keramidas G. Changes in magnitude of relative cerebri during the application of external forces on the frontal bone of an embalmed cadaver. *PT Forum*. 1991;10(10).

Kubovy M. *The Psychology of Perspective and Renaissance Art*. London: Cambridge University Press; 1986.

Lauer TQ. *Phenomenology and the Crises of Philosophy*. New York, NY: Harper & Row; 1965.

LeGuin UK. *The Earthsea Trilogy*. New York, NY: Bantam; 1968.

Levine P. The body as healer: a revisioning of trauma and anxiety. *Somatics*. 1990;8(1).

Lewit K. The functional approach. *The Journal of Orthopaedic Medicine*. 1994;16(3).

Malone T, Malone P. *The Art of Intimacy*. New York, NY: Prentice Hall; 1987.

Manheim C, Lavett D. *Craniosacral Therapy and Somato-Emotional Release*. Thorofare, NJ: SLACK Inc; 1989:61-62.

Meade M. *The Rag and Bone Shop of the Heart*. New York, NY: Harper Collins; 1992.

Milam L. *Crip Zen: A Manual for Survivors*. Mho and Mho Works; 1993.

Montagu A. *Touching: The Human Significance of the Skin*. New York, NY: Harper & Row; 1968.

Morelli M, Seaboune D, Sullivan S. Changes in H-reflex amplitude during massage of triceps surae in healthy subjects. *JOSPT*. 1990;12(2).

Morris D. *The Culture of Pain*. Berkeley, Calif: University of California Press; 1991.

Moyne J, Barks C. *Open Secret—Versions of Rumi*. Putney, Vt: Threshold Books; 1984.

Naumovski M. *Behind the eyes: the speaking of myopia*. Master's thesis.

New York Times Magazine. 1989;Dec 31.

Newton M, Waddell G. Trunk strength testing with iso-machines. *Spine*. 1993;18(7).

Orstein R. *Psychology of Consciousness*. New York, NY: Penguin; 1970.

Pearson C. *Awakening the Heroes Within*. New York, NY: Harper Collins; 1991.

Peck C. Reflections on the edge. *The Yoga Journal*. 1991;Sept/Oct.

Philosopher turned somatic educator: an interview with Jeffrey Maitland. *Massage Therapy Journal*. 1992;Spring.

Potter, Rothstein J. Intertester reliability for selected clinical tests of the sacroiliac joint. *Physical Therapy*. 1985;Nov.

PT Bulletin. 1994;Jul 27.

Quincey P. Why we are unmoved as oceans ebb and flow. *Skeptical Inquirer*. 1994;18(5):509-515.

Rosenfeld J. *The Invention of Memory*. New York, NY: Basic Books; 1988.

Rothman M. Myths about science...and belief in the paranormal. *Skeptical Inquirer*. 1989;Fall.

Rothstein J. *APTA Journal*. 1990;Aug. Editorial.

Sachs F. The intimate sense: understanding the mechanics of touch. *The Sciences*. 1988;Jan/Feb.

Sacks O. *A Leg to Stand On*. New York, NY: Summit Books; 1984.

Sacks O. *Awakenings*. New York, NY: EP Dutton; 1974.

Sacks O. *Migraine*. Berkeley, Calif: University of California Press.

Sacks O. *Seeing Voices, A Journey Into the World of the Deaf*. Berkeley, Calif: University of California Press; 1989.

Sacks O. *The Man Who Mistook His Wife for a Hat*. Magnolia, Mass: Peter Smith; 1992.

Sagan C. *The Dragons of Eden*. New York, NY: Random House; 1977.

Selzer R. *Mortal Lessons: Notes on the Art of Surgery*. New York, NY: Simon & Schuster; 1974.

Simeons ATW. *Man's Presumptuous Brain*. New York, NY: Dutton; 1961.

Springer S, Deutsch G. *Left Brain, Right Brain*. New York, NY: Freeman & Co; 1985:237-288.

Stafford W. *Stories That Could Be True*. 1977.

Stoll C. *Silicon Snake Oil: Second Thoughts on the Information Highway*. New York, NY: Doubleday; 1995

Strauch R. *The Reality Illusion*. Barrytown, NY: Station Hill; 1983.

Thomas L. On the uncertainty of science. *Harvard Magazine*. 1980;Sept/Oct.

Threlkeld AJ. The effect of manual therapy on connective tissue. *APTA Journal*. 1992;72(12).

Toombs SK. *The Meaning of Illness: A Phenomenological Account of the Different Perspectives of Physician and Patient*. Dordiecht: Kluwer; 1992.

Ventura M. Possibilities of ritual. *LA Weekly*. 1992;Jan 17.

Whyte D. Out on the ocean. *Songs for Coming Home*. Many Rivers Press; 1989.

Whyte D. *The Heart Aroused*. New York, NY: Doubleday; 1994.

Whyte D. *The Poetry of David Whyte*. Langly, Wash: Many Rivers Press.

SUGGESTED READING

Briggs J, Peat F. *Turbulent Mirror*. New York, NY: Harper & Row; 1989.

Donaldson OF. Chrysanthemum swords: towards an understanding of play as a universal martial art. *Somatics*. 1985-1986;5(3).

Dorko BL A simple test of autonomic balance. *PT Forum*. 1989;8(28).

Dorko BL. Adaptive potential: a new concept in pain of mechanical origin. *PT Forum*. 1988;7(29).

Dorko BL. *Fractal Geometry and Manual Care*. Available from the author.

Dorko BL. Juggling courageously. *Jugglers World*. 1992;Spring.

Dorko BL. Palpatory diagnoses and the irritative nerve lesion. *PT Forum*. 1989;8(13).

Dorko BL. Persistent pain and underlying processes. *PT Forum*. 1988;7(25).

Dorko BL. The use of simple contact. *PT Forum*. 1988;7(16).

Dorko BL. The use of somatic philosophy in the practice of physical therapy. *PT Forum*. 1989;8(3).

Gellhorn E. *Autonomic-Somatic Integrations: Physiologic Basis and Clinical Implications*. Minneapolis, Minn: University of Minnesota Press; 1967.

Goldberger A, et al. Chaos and fractals in human physiology. *Scientific American*. 1990;Feb.

Herbert M. Ecofeminist science and the physiology of the living body. *Somatics*. 1990;7(4).

Jayson MI, ed. *The Lumbar Spine and Back Pain*. 4th ed. New York, NY: Churchill Livingstone; 1992.

Lipsitz L, et al. Loss of "complexity" in aging potential applications of fractals and chaos theory to senescence. *JAMA*. 267(13).

Mindell A. *River's Way*. London: Rutledge and Kegan Paul Ltd; 1985.

Morris D. *Primate Ethology*. Wedenfield and Nicolson; 1967.

Pema C. Abandon any hope of fruition. *Pilgrimage*. 1994;20(2).

Sachs F. The intimate sense: understanding the mechanics of touch. *The Sciences*. 1988;Jan/Feb.

Scott A. The solitary wave. *The Sciences*. 1990;Mar/Apr.

The mathematics of human life. *US News and World Report*. 1993;Jun 14.